Fifth Edition

Baby & Me

The Essential Guide to Pregnancy and Newborn Care

Deborah D. Stewart
Jenny B. Harvey

Illustrated by Christine Thomas

Bull Publishing Company
Boulder, Colorado

Bull Publishing Company
P.O. Box 1377
Boulder, CO 80306
Phone: 800-676-2855
www.bullpub.com

Library of Congress Cataloging-in-Publication Data
Stewart, Deborah D.
  Baby & me : guide to pregnancy and newborn care / written by Deborah D. Stewart, Jenny B. Harvey; illustrated by Christine Thomas. — 5th ed.
    p. cm.
  Includes bibliographic references and index.
  ISBN 978-1-936693-76-4
  1. Pregnancy—Popular works. 2. Childbirth—Popular works.
  I. Title. II. Title: Baby and me.

Additional CIP data can be found at :

https://www.bullpub.com/downloads

Printed in U.S.A.

19 18 17 16   10 9 8 7 6 5 4 3 2

Design and production by Dovetail Publishing Services
Cover design by Shannon Bodie, Lightbourne Images

From Deborah to my second grandson, Charlie McCleary, now 8, and to my dearest late husband, Mike Gold, who provided constant encouragement and support.

From Jenny to James (MTIL), without whom I could not have been a part of this book, and to Violet Louise, who will always be my baby.

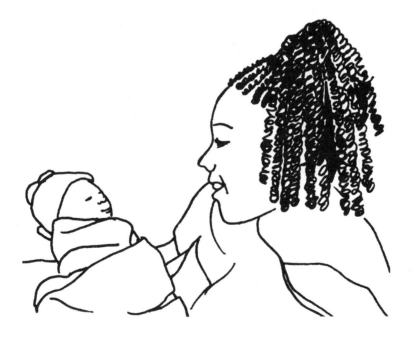

A note to you from Deborah . . .

My goal for *Baby & Me* for over 22 years and five editions has been to help parents stay healthy and happy during pregnancy and keep their newborn baby healthy. The more you can do to prevent health problems the better, for yourself and your baby. Here you will find basic information about pregnancy, birth, and baby care in an easy-to-use form. You will also find sources you can trust for more detailed information when you need it.

Good health is one of the best gifts you, as a parent, can give a child. I hope *Baby & Me* will encourage you to do all you can for your child. Caring for yourself and your baby is a big task. You deserve plenty of help to make it easier.

Best wishes to you and your baby! I hope you will enjoy this special time in your life. Your body is doing an amazing job. It has the power to grow and protect new life.

Deborah Davis Stewart, BA
Portland, Oregon

A note to you from Jenny . . .

Getting ready to have a baby is a big deal, and becoming a family is an even bigger deal! There is a lot to learn and make decisions about. Families come in all sizes, shapes, colors, and styles. My goal for *Baby & Me* is to give you information that you can use to make healthy choices that feel right for you and your family.

Taking care of yourself and your baby during pregnancy can help you worry less and enjoy more. Being prepared for your baby's birth can help you feel strong and calm. Talking to the people in your life who can help and support you can bring you closer together. All of this gives your baby a strong start to a good and healthy life!

Wishing you my keys to parenthood: strength, peace, sleep, patience, and lots of laughter!

Jenny Burris Harvey, BA
Seattle, Washington

Acknowledgments

This edition, the fifth, is a complete revision, not just a basic update. It went through a very thorough review process, so many of the reviewers put in more time and energy than we originally asked of them. We give our heartfelt thanks to all of these professionals. Their enthusiasm about *Baby & Me* and dedication to communicating the key information about prenatal and infant health in an easily understandable way has been boundless.

Barbara C. Decker, HBCE, CLD(CAPPA), Certified Prenatal Bonding Facilitator (BA & GPE): *www.soulofbirthing.com*

Melinda Ferguson, CD(DONA), PCD(DONA), PDT(DONA)

Debra Golden, RN, BSN, MS: Over 30 years of nursing and public health program management experience in maternal and child health, Alaska

Betsy Hayford, CNM: Affiliated with Legacy Emanuel Hospital, Portland, OR, for 20 years practicing midwifery and caring for families; now at Oregon Health Sciences University

Benjamin D. Hoffman, MD FAAP: Professor of Pediatrics, Oregon Health and Science University

Kim James, BDT(DONA), ICCE, LCCE

Elias Kass, ND, LM, CPM: Midwife and naturopathic doctor specializing in the care of babies and children, practicing at One Sky Family Medicine, Seattle, WA

Joy MacTavish-Unten, MA, IBCLC, RLC, ICCE: Owner, Sound Breastfeeding; Adjunct Faculty, The Simkin Center for Allied Birth Vocations, Bastyr University; Instructor, Great Starts, a program of Parent Trust for Washington Children

Lisa Meuleman, BSN: Public Health Nurse

Sharon Muza, BSc., CD(DONA), BDT(DONA), LCCE, FACCE: *sharonmuza.com*

Marni B. Port, MSW: Child & Teen Services Manager, Parent Trust for Washington Children

Maricela Vega, RN-BSN, RHIT: Perinatal Nurse, Mercy Hospital and Medical Center, Chicago, IL

Kathy Wilson, CCCE, CPD, IMPI Certified Sleep Consultant: H.U.G. Teacher, Tranquility Postpartum Support, *www.fourthtrimester.com*

And to the other professionals who shared their insight on infant care and safety, we thank you for helping us to make this edition of *Baby & Me* as up to date and helpful as possible.

Please note

This book should not be the only guide you use to care for yourself and your unborn child. Your doctor or midwife and other medical professionals are trained to help you take care of yourself. Please consult those who know your special needs.

Contents

Using this book   **xi**

   This book is yours!   xiii

   Sharing with partners, other family members   xiii

   Traditions in birth and baby care   xiii

   The words we use   xiv

   Medical words   xiv

1   **Get Ready for Pregnancy**   **1**

   Preparing your body for a baby   2

   Healthy habits   3

   For partners   6

2   **You're Pregnant—What's Next?**   **7**

   Your changing body   7

   Practical things to think about   10

   Tips for partners   13

3   **Keeping Your Body Healthy**   **15**

   Building healthy habits   17

   Germs and your unborn baby   25

   Hidden dangers, poisons   26

   Relax more, worry less   30

   Tips for partners   31

4   **What You Eat, Drink, and Breathe**   **33**

   Good Food: Giving Baby the Best   34

   Food warnings   41

   Preparing food safely   42

   Dangers for baby   44

   Tips for partners   49

5   Health Care for You and Baby   51

Choices in prenatal care and your birth   52

Plan ahead: care for baby   59

Tips for partners   60

6   Plan Ahead for Birth and Baby   61

Childbirth   62

Time off from work   65

Start learning about baby care   65

Things you and baby will need   67

Tips for partners   74

7   Your 9 Months to Get Ready   75

Trimesters, months, and weeks   76

Weeks 1 through 12   78

Warning signs—Emergency   83

Healthy habits   87

Partner abuse in pregnancy   88

Common worries   89

Warning signs of miscarriage   90

Tips for partners   93

Month-to-month checkups   94

8   Second Trimester: Months 4, 5, and 6   99

Weeks 13 to 28   99

Exercises for you now   102

Sex in pregnancy   104

Common problems   105

Medical things to know   108

Warning signs—Preterm labor   110

Tips for partners   111

Month-to-month checkups   112

9   Third Trimester: Months 7, 8, and 9   115

29 to 40 weeks   115

Third trimester basics   118

Warning signs—High blood pressure   120

Your body gets ready for labor   122
Your birth plan   126
Tips for partners   127
Month-to-month checkups   128

10   Your Baby's Birth   137
How birth happens naturally   140
STAGE 1: Labor   144
STAGE 2: The birth of your baby   149
STAGES 3 and 4: Tips for birth partners   151
Other Things to Know about Birth   152
Baby's Birth Day   162

11   Caring for Your New Baby   163
New baby's health   164
The first day   166
The first weeks at home   172
If your baby needs special care   178
Tips for partners   179

12   Feeding Your New Baby   181
Basics of feeding   182
Breastfeeding: Getting started   184
Going back to work or school   192
Feeding with a bottle   193
Tips for partners   196

13   Getting to Know Your Baby   197
A good start for the family   198
Understanding your new baby   200
Helping baby sleep   207
When baby cries   208
Tips for partners   211

14   Keeping Your Baby Safe   213
Sleep safety: SIDS and suffocation   214
Car seats for baby on the go   217

Other safety measures 222

Tips for partners 226

15 Keeping Your Baby Healthy 227

Ways to keep baby healthy 228

Well-baby checkups 229

Vaccines fight deadly diseases 230

When baby gets sick 235

Warning signs—Serious illness 236

Warning—Giving antibiotics 239

Tips for partners 240

Your baby's first checkups 241

16 Taking Care of Yourself 243

What to expect as your body heals 244

Warning signs—First weeks after delivery 245

Your own six-week checkup 248

Sex after baby 248

How are you feeling? 250

Warning signs—Mood disorders 251

Tips for partners 253

Affirmations for parents 254

17 Resources to Help You 255

Help where you live 256

Websites and national resources 257

Women's health resources 257

Baby-care resources 259

Books to keep handy 261

Glossary: Words to know 263

Index 269

Using This Book

If you are pregnant or thinking of getting pregnant, taking care of yourself now is the most important thing you can do to have a healthy, happy baby. This book can help. Take a quick look all the way through it. Then read the chapters again, as your pregnancy moves along.

This book is yours!

Keep it handy and use it often. Highlight or write in it as much as you like. Mark pages you want to go back to. Use the notes pages to keep track of how you feel, questions you have, or things your provider says that you want to remember.

Partners, grandparents, other family members

This book isn't just for moms. Dads, moms, and other partners go through huge changes when getting ready for baby, too. Partners will play a big part in a baby's life, from pregnancy on. So we have created a special place at the end of each chapter with tips just for them. We hope you will share these partner tips, and the rest of the book, with them.

Grandparents and other relatives may play a big role in caring for their grandbabies. Share this book with them. We hope it will help them catch up on the latest best practices in pregnancy, birth, and baby care. Sharing this book may help you talk with them about how they can be a part of this new life.

Traditions in birth and baby care

The advice in this book may be different from what your family or your people have done in the past. Sometimes, women tell you how things should be done simply because that's how they did them. Other times, it is cultural tradition that things are done a certain way. For example, in some cultures, certain foods are not eaten during pregnancy. In others, the baby's father usually does not take part in the birth.

There are many ways to good health, and family values are important. The ideas in this book, which come from the most current science, will give you and your baby a healthy start. If you wish to do something different, talk about it with your doctor, nurse, or midwife. Tell them your reasons or concerns. Listen to what they say. Then decide what you feel is best for you and your baby.

The words we use

All families, parents, and babies are unique. In this book, we have tried to welcome and include all people. We especially want you to know that this book is for you, no matter what age you are, if you have a partner or not, and no matter what gender you or your partner may be.

We will take turns saying "mom" and "parent," "dad" and "partner." But, most of the time, what we cover is meant to be true for any birthing person and any kind of partner or support person.

We will take turns using "he" and "she" when we talk about babies. But, what we cover will almost always be true for any baby. The same thing goes for how we use "he" and "she" for doctors, nurses, and midwives.

Medical words

There are many different names for medical people who might care for you. We often will use "healthcare provider" or just "provider" instead of "doctor, midwife, or nurse" in this book.

Medical talk can be confusing. We have tried to use words that are easy to understand. You will find it helpful to learn some medical words, since your provider may use them a lot. When you see a word marked with a star like this*, you can see what it means at the side of that page. Meanings of many words you will need to know are in the glossary at the end of Chapter 17.

Chapter 1

Get Ready for Pregnancy

Preparing your body for a baby

Start now to make sure your body is a healthy home for a baby.
Before you get pregnant is the best time to get your body ready.
But it's never too soon or too late to start taking care of yourself.
The food you eat, the air you breathe, and the things you do all
affect how your baby will grow.

Many women get pregnant when they don't expect it.
Sometimes they don't know for a few months. Even if a woman is
trying to get pregnant, most don't know for a week or two. Yet
these early weeks are when special parts of baby's body form.

Living your life as if you might be pregnant is wise.

Getting healthy before pregnancy

A baby's body starts to form right away after pregnancy begins.
This happens before you know you are pregnant. So being healthy
now means your unborn baby will have the best chance of being

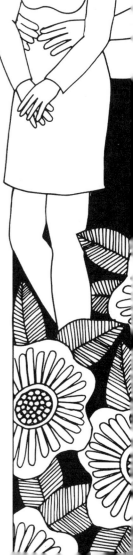

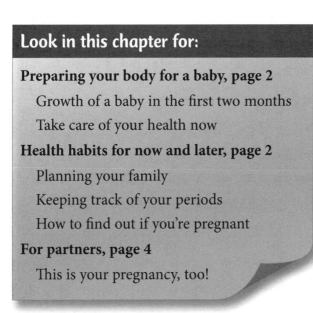

Look in this chapter for:

Preparing your body for a baby, page 2

    Growth of a baby in the first two months

    Take care of your health now

Health habits for now and later, page 2

    Planning your family

    Keeping track of your periods

    How to find out if you're pregnant

For partners, page 4

    This is your pregnancy, too!

Baby's growth in the first two months (life size)

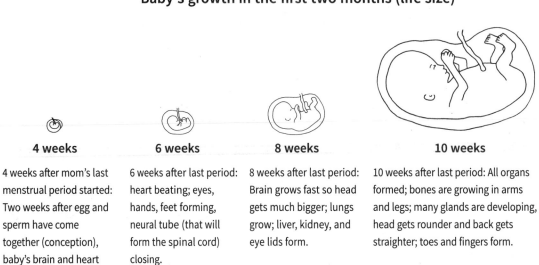

| **4 weeks** | **6 weeks** | **8 weeks** | **10 weeks** |

4 weeks after mom's last menstrual period started: Two weeks after egg and sperm have come together (conception), baby's brain and heart are forming. Baby's body has a front and back, top and bottom.

6 weeks after last period: heart beating; eyes, hands, feet forming, neural tube (that will form the spinal cord) closing.

8 weeks after last period: Brain grows fast so head gets much bigger; lungs grow; liver, kidney, and eye lids form.

10 weeks after last period: All organs formed; bones are growing in arms and legs; many glands are developing, head gets rounder and back gets straighter; toes and fingers form.

healthy, too. Problems caused by mom's poor health now can affect a child all through life. Share this fact with your friends.

These life-sized drawings show the growth of the baby in the first months. All the most important parts start growing then.

Take care of your health now

"It's amazing . . . I had no idea how fast a baby starts developing. Nobody told me how careful I should be before I got pregnant."

Good health now can prevent many health problems for you and your baby later. Every mom wants the best for her baby. It's better to be careful now than wish later you had done things differently.

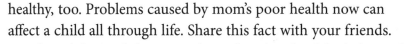

- ◆ Take a vitamin pill with folate (or folic acid) in it every day. Folate helps baby's brain and spinal cord grow right.
- ◆ Stop using alcohol, tobacco, pot, or other drugs. Any time you smoke, drink alcohol, or use drugs, a baby growing inside would get some too.
- ◆ Get health problems under control. Diabetes and high blood pressure are two common problems. Get care for them now.
- ◆ Stay away from chemicals or animal feces (poop) that can be harmful.

◆ Ask your health care provider* if any medicines or drugs you take could affect a baby if you get pregnant.

◆ Get health insurance if you don't have it already.

See Chapters 3, 4, and 5 to learn more.

*Health care provider:
A professional who cares for people's health.

Health habits for now and later

Planning your family is part of good health

Controlling when you get pregnant is part of taking care of your body. Any time you have sex, even once, you could get pregnant. Talk to your partner about birth control (contraception) before you have sex. A woman needs to use effective birth control every time so you won't get pregnant.

Talk to your partner before you stop using birth control. Make sure you both are really ready to have a baby. You will all have a better life if you start out healthy. See Chapter 16 to learn more about kinds of birth control you can trust.

A visit to your doctor or nurse

Before you get pregnant, visit your doctor, nurse, or midwife. They can tell you how to take the best care of yourself now. If you don't have a health care provider, now is a good time to get one. (See Chapter 5.)

Talk to them about the six things listed above. Get advice about things that worry you, like your age, weight, or health problems. If someone in your family has a genetic disease, ask about genetic counseling.

Keep track of your periods

Before you get pregnant, keep track of your menstrual periods (monthly cycle or flow). This helps you know when your period is late. Knowing when your last period started will help you and your provider figure out when your baby will be born (your due date).

Use a calendar to keep track of your period each month. Put an X on each day you have bleeding. This helps you know how long your periods last and how far apart they come.

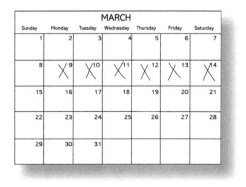

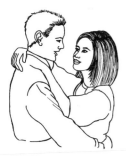

You and your partner—Building a team

Partners play a big role in a healthy pregnancy. It's important to support each other. Talk with your partner about starting healthy habits together. For example, start eating healthier foods and help each other stop smoking.

*Fertility:
Ability to get
pregnant.

Some women get pregnant right away. Others have to try for a while. If you have a hard time getting pregnant, see your provider again. There are many things that can help your fertility*. Ask what you and your partner can do. Sometimes simple things make a big difference. You may also ask about fertility care. Know your options so you can choose what is best for you.

How do I know if I'm pregnant?

Here are the first main signs of pregnancy:

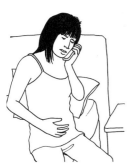

- ◆ Late period or no period at all
- ◆ Tiredness
- ◆ Sore, swollen breasts
- ◆ Upset stomach

If your period is late and you have any other of these signs, you might be pregnant. Get a pregnancy test. **Start taking care of yourself as if you were pregnant.**

A positive pregnancy test means you are pregnant. If you have a positive test, it's time to see a doctor, nurse, or midwife. Make an appointment right away. You could also go to your local health clinic.

How do I get a pregnancy test?

You can buy a pregnancy test to use at home. Also, a test can be done at a clinic or your doctor, nurse, or midwife's office. Some clinics, like Planned Parenthood, may have free pregnancy tests.

Home pregnancy tests check your urine (pee) for pregnancy hormones. Most drug stores or grocery stores have them. You don't need a prescription. They can be used very soon after you miss your period. A positive test means you're pregnant.

A negative test could mean that you aren't pregnant.It also could mean that you took the test too soon. Wait a week and take another test. Or, see your provider.

A test in the office or clinic checks your blood for pregnancy hormones. These tests can be done even before you miss a period. They are very accurate. You may also have an ultrasound* if your period is more than a few weeks late.

If you're not pregnant but still have no period, call your provider. This can be a sign of health problems.

*Ultrasound:
A tool to look at baby inside your uterus. A wand is moved around on your belly. Pictures show on the screen.

What do I do after I take the test?

Start taking extra care of your body. Read Chapters 2, 3, and 4. Look ahead at the rest of the book. It will take you through your pregnancy and beyond birth.

If you are not pregnant, now is a good time to make some changes. Use all you learned in this chapter to get your body healthy before you do get pregnant. If you don't want to get pregnant, use birth control every time you have sex. If you're afraid the kind you use is not going to work, use another kind. See Chapter 16 to learn more.

If you are pregnant, make an appointment with your doctor, nurse, or midwife. Tell them you are pregnant when you call. And start taking care of yourself.

If you are not sure you are ready to be a parent, talk with someone you trust right away. Ask a social worker, doctor, nurse, school counselor, or midwife about the different options you might have. Whatever you choose to do, be sure to take good care of your health now.

If you are sure you're ready to be pregnant, the provider will likely want to see you 1 to 2 months after your first missed period. At that time, the baby is big enough to show on an ultrasound.

Now is the time to explore the life that lies ahead for you and your future child. Start by reading Chapter 2 and beyond.

Partners: This is your pregnancy, too!

You can play a key part in this pregnancy. Being involved is not just a responsibility as a parent but also can be interesting and even joyful.

At the end of each chapter, you will find a short part with tips you can use every month. We hope you will check these out as your baby grows and becomes more real.

This may be the first time you think much about how babies grow. The natural growth and birth of a baby is amazing. It seems like magic but it isn't. Reading the whole book will help you understand this special event.

Chapter 2

You're Pregnant—What's Next?

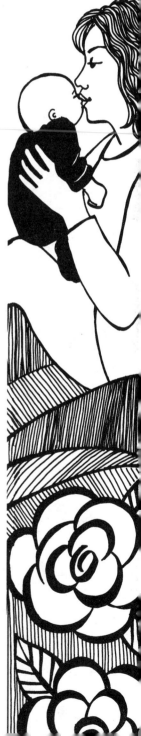

Being pregnant can make you feel both excited and scared. Most people have mixed feelings—and a lot of questions.

How will a baby change my life?

What will childbirth be like?

Will my baby be healthy?

Will I be a good parent?

It can be hard not knowing what life is going to be like later. Making some changes now can help make it easier down the road. Now is the time to learn about making a healthy life for you and your unborn baby.

What's happening to me?

Your body is starting to change in many ways before your belly begins to show. You may start to feel different right away.

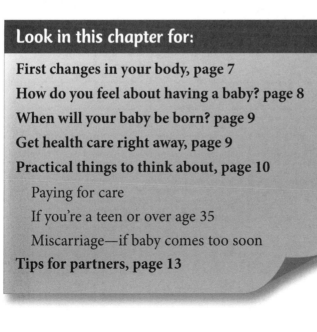

Look in this chapter for:

First changes in your body, page 7

How do you feel about having a baby? page 8

When will your baby be born? page 9

Get health care right away, page 9

Practical things to think about, page 10

Paying for care

If you're a teen or over age 35

Miscarriage—if baby comes too soon

Tips for partners, page 13

First changes in your body

- You will have no period. You're already about two weeks pregnant when you miss your first period!
- Your breasts may swell and hurt.
- You may feel more tired than usual.
- You may feel like throwing up (vomiting).
- You may need to urinate (pee) more often.
- Your mood may change often. You may feel sad one minute and very happy the next.

How do you feel about having a baby?

Check how you are feeling and write what you are thinking below:

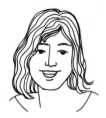

____ It's wonderful.

____ It feels strange.

____ It's hard to believe.

____ I don't feel ready to have a baby.

I am happy about_____

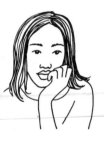

_____

_____

_____

I wonder about _____

_____

_____

_____

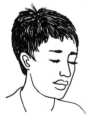

I am worried about_____

_____

_____

_____

Talk with your partner. Be honest and kind. If you are worried about something, say so. Talking together may help. Have your partner answer the questions on page 13. Then, share your answers with each other. It's a great way to start.

When will my baby be born?

Your "due date" is the best guess about when your baby will be born. Remember, babies don't always come on that date.

If you had unprotected sex only one time, you may know exactly when you got pregnant. To find the due date, use a calandar to count 38 weeks from the date you had sex.

If you know the date your last period started, you can estimate the date. A baby takes about 40 weeks to grow after your last period began. Here's how to figure it out. (Write in dates below.)

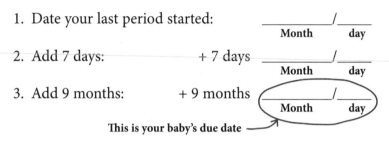

1. Date your last period started: _____/_____
                                      Month   day

2. Add 7 days: + 7 days   _____/_____
                                      Month   day

3. Add 9 months: + 9 months   ⟨_____/_____⟩
                                      Month   day

This is your baby's due date ——→

If you don't know when your last period started, your provider can find the due date. Using an ultrasound, they can see how big your uterus* is and how big your baby is. This will tell them how long you've been pregnant. Then they can tell you when your baby may be born.

*Uterus:
The part of the body where an unborn baby grows. Also called the womb.

Most babies come between two weeks before and two weeks after their due dates. **Labor will start when your baby and your body are ready. A baby born at least 39 weeks after your last period is called full-term.** Be ready in case your baby comes a few weeks early. But be patient in case your baby comes a little later.

Get health care right away

You should see a doctor or midwife right away. You may be thrilled to be pregnant or scared that you are not ready to have a baby. In any case, they can give you the help and care you need.

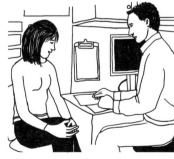

See Chapter 5 for different kinds of health care providers for pregnancy. It will also tell you what your first prenatal visit* will be like.

*Prenatal visits:
Checkups during pregnancy to keep you and your baby safe and healthy.

Practical things to think about

Paying for care

Find out how to pay for prenatal care and child birth. Ask your insurance, employer, or health clinic. How much will be covered? What will you have to pay for yourself? What choices do you have for care?

If you don't have health insurance, get signed up now. (See Chapter 5.)

Money to raise a baby

Having a family costs money. Start saving and planning as soon as you know you're pregnant. Find out what resources are in your area for pregnant women. Your local health clinic, family center, library, or food bank is a good place to start to find help. Many churches and community centers offer money planning help, too. (See the list in Chapter 17.) You can still be a wonderful parent, even if you don't have a lot of money.

Think ahead. Do you have a good job? Will you be able to keep it? Can you afford child care? Many of these places can help you come up with a plan, go back to school, or look for a good job. Some can even give you clothes, tips, and child care for job interviews. The more prepared you feel, the less worried you will be.

If you don't have a partner

Remember, a family can be any small group who share their lives and support each other with love.

You don't have to go through this alone. Close friends and family can be great support during pregnancy and birth. Find a few people who you can count on to listen and help you feel safe and loved. Some health clinics have support groups or prenatal classes for single moms-to-be.

You'll also want to take some time to think about who will be with you when your baby is born. Maybe a family member or a friend. You could also find out about low-cost doulas* in your area. Having support during pregnancy, birth, and after is very important.

*Doula:
a person trained to give comfort and support to women during and after birth. Not a medical professional but often very helpful.

If you're a teen

These are big changes happening in your life. You can be a great parent to your child. You'll have to make serious choices and new plans. It may feel hard to know what is best. Just be sure to get help soon, not put it off too long.

As a teen, you're more likely than an adult to have some health problems during pregnancy. You're more likely to have a baby that is born too soon or very small. The best way to have a healthy baby is to start getting prenatal care as soon as you think you might be pregnant. Then be sure to go to all of your appointments.

Talk to someone you trust about what's happening. People you might turn to:

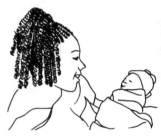

- your parents or relatives

- a close friend or a close friend's mom or dad

- the school nurse or counselor

- your regular doctor or nurse

- someone at your place of worship

Young parents may also have a hard time with money, finding a place to live, and finishing school. Many health clinics and family centers have groups or social workers to help you figure things out and make a plan.

If you're over age 35

There is no exact age when you are "too old to have a baby." Every woman is different. However, after 35, there are a few more problems that could happen to mom and baby.

High blood pressure and diabetes are more likely for older moms-to-be. Miscarriage (see below) and stillbirth* are a bit more common as mom gets older. There is also more of a chance that baby will have birth defects. Talk with your provider about how to make sure you and baby are as healthy as possible.

*Stillbirth:
A baby born after 20 weeks with no signs of life.

Miscarriage—When baby comes too soon

Some pregnancies end in the first 20 weeks, before the baby can live outside the uterus. This is called a miscarriage. Most happen in the first 7 weeks of pregnancy. It can happen before you even know you're pregnant. In most cases there is no way to stop it.

In case they miscarry, some women wait until after the first trimester to tell people they're pregnant. Other women only tell close friends at first. This way, they have some privacy but also get support if they miscarry. Think about what feels right for you before you tell the world your news.

What is a miscarriage like?

The common signs of miscarriage are:

- cramps (like period cramps)
- bleeding or a bloody blob from your vagina
- belly pain
- low back pain

Some of these signs could be normal in early pregnancy. But, just in case, it's best to call your provider. (For more about miscarriage, see the end of Chapter 7.)

Why does miscarriage happen?

In most cases, the cause is never known. Most happen because the baby isn't growing right. It can also happen because of problems with the mom's body.

It can be very emotional to miscarry. You may feel sad, scared, or even relieved. It's okay to have a lot of feelings about it. Talk to someone and share what happened. You could tell your partner, or a trusted friend or relative. You may want to talk to your doctor, midwife, a counselor, or someone from your clinic or place of worship. You might find a support group with others who have been through this. Remember that most women who miscarry can have a healthy pregnancy later.

Tips for partners

Getting pregnant changes your life, too! Both your partner and your unborn baby need you during this special time. There are many ways to be a good partner and a good parent, from the start.

- ◆ Give mom and baby your love and support. You'll have lots of feelings about having a baby. Be gentle and kind.

- ◆ Put your hand on your partner's belly. Tell your baby that you will try your best to be a good parent.

- ◆ Learn about pregnancy, birth, and baby care. Getting ready now can make things easier later.

- ◆ Help her live a healthy life. Take care of yourself and your partner to give baby the best start in life.

- ◆ Think ahead. Your lives change with a baby. Make plans for your home, job, money, and future.

Partners may have mixed feelings

Mixed feelings of happiness and worry are OK. Check below the feelings that you have, or write in your thoughts:

____ It's wonderful.

____ It feels strange.

____ It's hard to believe.

____ I don't feel ready to help care for a baby.

As a partner, I am happy about _____

_____

_____

_____

I am worried about _____

_____

_____

_____

I am a little bit afraid of _____

_____

_____

_____

Talk with your pregnant partner. Be honest and kind. Tell her if you are worried about something. Talking may help. Ask her how she answered these questions. It's important to share your feelings with each other. Remember, you will get used to this new life during the next 9 months.

Your lifestyle partnership:

- Encourage your baby's mom to eat healthy foods. Try to eat well yourself.

- Help her avoid smoking, drinking alcohol, or taking any other drugs. Find other things to do together. Plan visits with friends, listen to relaxing music, or take her for a picnic.

- If you smoke, do so outside, away from your baby's mom. Second-hand smoke or vapor from your cigarettes can affect your unborn baby.

- Take walks and do prenatal exercises with your partner.

- Share home chores, like laundry, cooking, and cleaning.

Take part in mom's health care:

"We could see the baby moving and his heart beating on the ultrasound! It finally felt real to me. I was finally as excited as she was."

—A new dad

- Find out as much as you can about pregnancy and being a parent.

- Offer to go with your partner to prenatal visits.

- Go to childbirth classes. You will learn what to expect and how to help during birth.

- Put your hand on her belly to feel your growing baby move inside.

Your feelings and concern for mom's feelings:

- Avoid making fun of or judging your partner's changing body. Many women worry about how their bodies look. Her weight gain is for her baby's health.

- Talk over your feelings about becoming parents. Let her know about your excitement and concerns. Listen to her feelings. Give her an extra hug if she is feeling unhappy.

- Talk to your unborn baby. A baby in the uterus can hear voices in the months before he's born. (Your baby may even know your voice when he is born.)

Chapter 3

Keeping Your Body Healthy

What you do every day is important for your baby's health—and your own. It's easy to say, "live a healthy life." But, do you know what that means and how to do it? This chapter can help.

Now you are pregnant, you have the best reason in the world for changing your habits. These habits are good for everyone. But, they are more important than ever during pregnancy.

I feel fine, so why do I need so many checkups?

Prenatal care is medical care for your pregnancy. You will have a lot of prenatal visits. These checkups help your health care provider learn how your baby and you are doing. He will look for health problems you can't feel.

If you and baby are both doing well, you will have one visit each month. In the last two months, you will have more checkups.

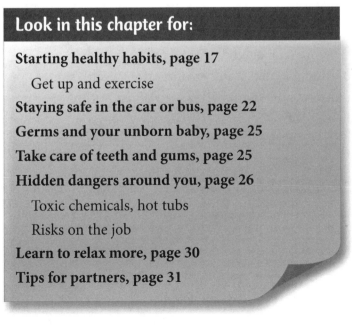

Look in this chapter for:

Starting healthy habits, page 17

   Get up and exercise

Staying safe in the car or bus, page 22

Germs and your unborn baby, page 25

Take care of teeth and gums, page 25

Hidden dangers around you, page 26

   Toxic chemicals, hot tubs

   Risks on the job

Learn to relax more, page 30

Tips for partners, page 31

Your provider will check:

◆ your baby's growth, heart rate, and movement

◆ how you feel and how your body is changing

◆ how much weight you've gained

◆ your blood pressure*

*Blood pressure:
The force of the blood pumped by the heart through your blood vessels. High blood pressure means the heart is working extra hard.

Most women have healthy babies. Regular visits help make this happen. Checkups can help catch problems early. Early treatment of any problems is best.

Your provider wants to hear your questions. What are you worried about? What do you want to know more about? Your prenatal visits are the best time to ask questions. As you go through this book, write down questions that you want to ask on the checkup pages. These are in Chapters 7, 8, and 9.

For more about prenatal visits and finding a provider, see Chapter 5.

Learning about healthy habits

Your health care provider is your best first source of information. But, there are many sources of health advice, like books, TV shows, websites, or people you know. Some of what you hear or read may not be true.

Some advice can be very confusing. You may hear good news one day about a product, food, or activity. The next day, some other source may say it is not healthy. Which advice can you believe?

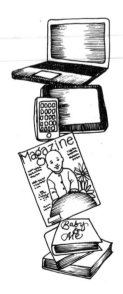

You are making a good start by using this book. It has been written using the newest information from health sources you can trust. Doctors, nurses, midwives, and others with proper training have reviewed it.

Here are questions to ask before you trust something new that you hear or read:

◆ Where did the information first come from (person, company, or organization)? Is it a source that you can trust? You can trust the national health organizations listed in Chapter 17.

◆ Are they trying to sell something?

◆ Is the report new? Look for a date on books or pamphlets. Some may be so old that they are out of date. But, news on

TV or the web may be so new that it hasn't really been proven.

♦ Have you asked your doctor or midwife about the advice you've heard? What do they tell you?

Start healthy habits right now

Your unborn baby is growing fast. Look back at the pictures of the very tiny baby in Chapter 1. All the main parts of the body (brain, spinal cord, and organs) are formed in the first two months. This is why you need to take care of yourself from the start of pregnancy.

The pictures below show how much your baby grows in the first four months. Even more amazing changes are taking place inside!

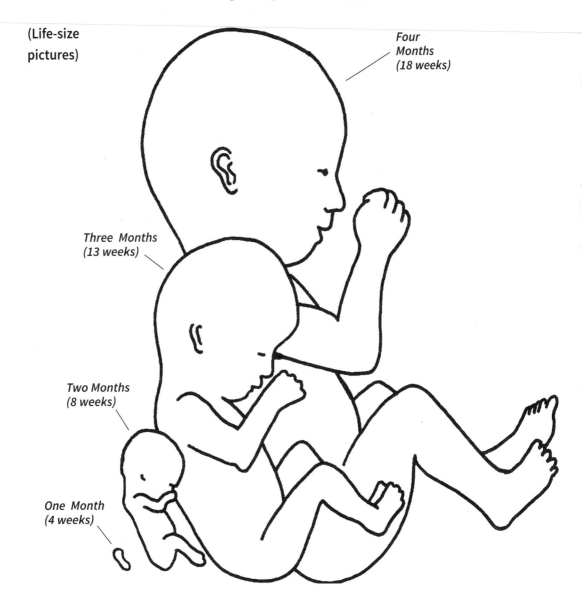

(Life-size pictures)

Four Months (18 weeks)

Three Months (13 weeks)

Two Months (8 weeks)

One Month (4 weeks)

How healthy are your habits now?

Most of us already have some habits that help an unborn baby. We also have other habits that could be unhealthy. Look at the list below. Try to be honest about how often you do them.

Healthy Habits	Yes	Some-times	No
I eat five or more servings of fruits and vegetables daily.			
I drink at least eight glasses of water and other liquids (not sodas) every day.			
I get about seven to eight hours of sleep every night.			
I exercise for about 30 minutes at least three times a week.			
I take some time to relax every day.			
I talk over my worries with others.			
I brush my teeth and floss daily.			
Unhealthy Habits	Yes	Some-times	No
I sit down for six or more hours straight each day.			
I smoke tobacco, e-cigarettes, marijuana.			
I drink beer, wine, wine coolers, or hard liquor.			
I take drugs that my doctor has not prescribed or that are illegal.			

Nobody's perfect, but you are making a good start!

Now write down the habits that you would like to change:

_____

_____

_____

_____

You may need help changing habits. Don't be shy about asking for help. That is the right thing to do for your baby.

Get up and move

Being active is good for both you and your growing baby. Exercise helps you get stronger, sleep better, and feel happier. If you have not exercised much before, check with your provider first.

Why should I make time for exercise?

Exercise may help you:

+ Stay at a healthy weight during and after pregnancy

+ Keep blood sugar and blood pressure normal

+ Reduce the chance of labor starting too early

+ Lessen back aches, hip pain, stiffness, swelling, and varicose veins*

+ Help avoid gas, constipation, even hemorrhoids*

Exercise doesn't just help your body get strong. It also helps you relax, cope with stress, and feel good about yourself. All of these things help you to be ready for labor and birth.

*Varicose veins: Swollen blue veins in your legs that can hurt.

*Hemorrhoids: Swollen veins in your bottom (anus) that may itch, bleed, or be sore.

What kinds of exercise are best?

Talk with your provider about what kinds of exercise he advises. If you don't already exercise, start with something easy like walking. Try to be active for 30 minutes at least three or four times a week.

+ Most activites are safe to keep doing while pregnant, but not all. Try to avoid things that are very bouncy. Don't do things that could make you fall, jump, or get hit in the belly.

+ Walking is one of the best exercises. It is good for your whole body. And, it's easy and free! Wear good walking shoes and bring a water bottle.

+ Swimming is great during pregnancy. It's good for your heart and helps calm swelling. Feeling so light in the water can also feel very good.

+ Exercise and gently stretch the core* of your body. This will help lessen back aches during pregnancy. It will make you strong for pushing in childbirth. You may be more flexible than normal, so be careful not to go too far.

*Core: Your tummy (abs) and back muscles.

- Prenatal yoga is good for your core. It also also helps you learn to relax. This will be very helpful when you are in labor.

Ways to make exercising easier

- Walk with a friend. Exercising together, you can get each other moving. It can make exercise less boring.
- You can exercise for 10 or 15 minutes several times a day. This can be easier for you than one longer session.
- Try an exercise class. Many hospitals, gyms, and community centers offer prenatal classes. There are walking and swimming groups for pregnant women.

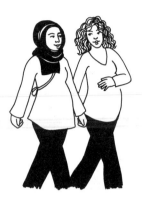

"I hate exercising. But when my friend and I started walking together, the time just flew by! It got me out the door twice a week and we talked about all kinds of things."

What else should I know about exercise?

- Drink plenty of water before, during, and after exercise.
- Exercise when it's cool outside. Try not to get too hot.
- Be extra careful if you live in high altitude, or where it gets very hot or very cold.
- Sit down and rest if you are uncomfortable, dizzy, too hot, or have trouble breathing.

STOP exercising and call your provider if you:

- Get dizzy or lightheaded often
- Have pain in your chest, belly, or legs
- Get a headache or have trouble seeing
- Have sudden swelling in your legs
- Feel contractions
- Have blood or fluid come from your vagina

Great exercises for your core*

Start strengthening your tummy and back right away. Many people don't do this before pregnancy, so their muscles need a lot of work. You can do these simple exercises when you are standing, sitting, or lying in bed.

Standing tall and straight

Standing with your belly hanging forward can make your back hurt. Standing up straight can lessen low-back pain. Walking straight also helps you feel good about yourself. Watch yourself do it in a big mirror the first time.

1. Wear comfortable shoes with a low heel. Stand sideways to the mirror. See how curved your low back is.

2. Now, pull your chin down and keep your ears right above your shoulders.

3. Take a deep breath and pull your shoulders back. Squeeze your shoulder blades down your back.

4. Let your breath out. Pull your tummy in. Keep your shoulders back. Check to see that your lower back is less curved.

5. Move back and forth a few times to get the feel for it.

See how your body looks different. Feel how your tummy and back muscles work together. Practice standing and walking this way. It will be good for you now and after baby comes, too.

One way to practice is to stand with your back to the wall and pull your back and shoulders back against the wall.

"Pelvic tilt" helps back pain

This makes your stomach muscles stronger and stretches your back. It can help you carry the extra weight without hurting your back.

1. Rest on hands and knees with your back straight.

2. Breathe in and pull your shoulders back. Lift your chest. Hold and count to five.

3. Breathe out while you tighten your tummy muscles. Pull your shoulders forward and arch your back like a cat.

4. Hold and count to five.

5. Breathe in again and pull your shoulders back. Flatten your back.

After the first four months, do this standing up.

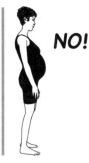

NO!

Does your back curve and belly hang out? This is a habit you can break.

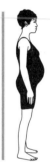

Get in the habit of standing straight and pulling in your belly.

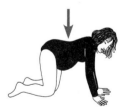

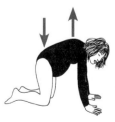

The pelvic tilt.

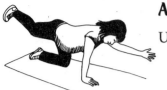

Arm and leg lift.

Arm and leg lifts

Use this exercise to strengthen your back.

1. Rest on hands and knees with your back straight. Pull in your belly.

2. Raise one arm straight out. Then raise the opposite leg straight out.

3. Hold and count to five.

4. Lower the arm and leg.

5. Raise the other arm and opposite leg. Count to five.

6. Repeat 10 times on each side.

Staying safe in the car or bus

You probably drive or ride in a car, van, pickup truck, or bus almost every day. Car travel seems so safe, but it's not. Driving to the grocery store, mall, or your job may be the most dangerous thing you do. It also is the biggest danger to your unborn baby.

Crashes are the most common cause of death and injury to young people. Most were not using seat belts. If you get hurt in a crash, your unborn baby will probably be hurt, too. Your body cannot protect your baby from all the forces of a crash. Even if you are not hurt, your baby could be.

All cars and some buses have seat belts. Using a seat belt makes you and your baby much safer. The seat belt keeps you from being thrown out in a crash. It also keeps you from being tossed around inside the car. Air bags add even more safety in serious crashes.

Do you ride safely? (check the things you always do)

____ I always use a seat belt, even in the back seat. If the bus has seat belts, I use them.

____ I have a car with air bags.

____ I say "no" to riding with a driver who has been drinking or using drugs.

____ If I need to text or answer a phone call, I stop the car first. I know both are distracting and often cause crashes. Using a hands-free phone isn't any safer.

Now work on getting better about the safety habits you have not been doing.

Wear your seat belt right

A seat belt that goes across your lap and shoulder is the safest kind. Use this kind whenever you can. It is important to fit the belt around your belly. Here's how:

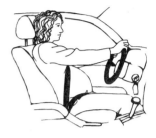

1. Push the lap part of the belt down under your belly. It should touch your thighs. Being below your belly keeps it from pushing on your uterus in a sudden stop or crash. To make the lap belt snug, pull up on the shoulder belt.

2. Put the shoulder belt over the middle of your shoulder, between your breasts and above your belly. Try adjusting the height at the top to help it fit well. Don't ever put the shoulder belt behind your back or under your arm. That could cause serious injury in a crash.

3. If you have a car with separate lap and shoulder belts, always buckle both of them. If it only has lap belts, buckle the belt down under your belly. Make it snug.

What about air bags?

All newer cars today have two front air bags, one in the steering wheel and the other in the dashboard. A front air bag works with the seat belt to protect you in a crash. It does not take the place of the seat belt. You need the seat belt to protect you and keep you in the car.

How to sit safely in a car with air bags:

- Sit back from the dashboard or steering wheel. Move your seat as far back as it can go.

- Keep your belly and chest at least 10 inches away from the dash or steering wheel, if you can.

- If your steering wheel tilts, aim it at your chest, not your head or belly.

- If you have a hard time reaching the pedals, try reclining the back. Then move the seat forward.

Most newer cars have side air bags, too. These may be in the doors or seats. Some seat belts also have air bags in the shoulder part. Check the car owner's manual for advice.

When it's not safe to drive

It's usually okay to drive during pregnancy. But, sometimes it's dangerous. Being very tired or feeling sick can make it hard to focus on driving. Even just having a lot on your mind can make you distracted.

Don't drive if you are dizzy, have a headache or vision problems. It's better not to drive if you don't have to.

If you are in a crash

Get checked out at an emergency room or doctor's office right away after any kind of crash. Do this even if you feel okay.

Be sure to tell the doctor you are pregnant. It's important to make sure your baby, uterus, placenta, and the rest of your body aren't hurt.

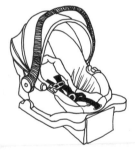

Baby will need a car seat

Right now your body and your seat belt protect your baby. But, she will need her own car seat (child safety seat) after birth. You will need to use it for every car ride. Car seats protect babies very well and are required by law in all states. (See Chapter 6 for how to choose a car seat. Read Chapter 14 for how to use it right.)

Safe sex still matters

It's nice not to have to worry about birth control while you're pregnant. But, pregnancy isn't the only thing that can happen during sex. You also may need protection against infections that spread through sex, often called STDs or STIs*. Any STD can be very harmful to your baby.

*STDs or STIs: Sexually transmitted diseases (STDs) are also called sexually transmitted infections (STIs). They include herpes, syphilis, gonorrhea, hepatitis B and C, chlamydia, and HIV.

Have STDs treated right away

Every pregnant woman should have tests for STDs at their first prenatal visit. If you think you may have an STD, be sure to say so when you go in. Most STDs can be treated during pregnancy. Some can't be cured, such as HIV and herpes. But, treatment can keep them from spreading to baby.

Prevent getting an STD

It's better to avoid getting an STD than have to cure one. The only ways to prevent STDs are:

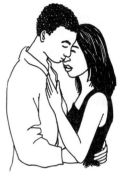

1. Have one sex partner who only has sex with you.

2. Use a condom every time you have sex. Other kinds of birth control do not protect you from STDs at all.

3. Do not have sex.

Germs and your unborn baby

It is never fun to get sick. But, getting sick while pregnant can be very hard and even dangerous for baby.

Easy ways to prevent sickness

People in good health get sick less than people who don't take care of themselves. Take care of yourself in all the ways talked about in this book. Also:

1. Avoid people who seem sick.

2. Wash hands often.

3. Get your **vaccines**. Get your flu shot and your pertussis (whooping cough) shot (Tdap). Talk to your provider about other vaccines you may want while you are pregnant.

Vaccines help keep you and your baby safe from dangerous illness.

4. Have those around you get their vaccines, too. This helps keep baby safe after birth, too.

If you do get sick

Ask your provider what kinds of symptoms you should call for. Watch out for fever, dehydration, rashes, or signs of infection. Ask your provider before taking any kind of medicine. Some medicines are not safe to take while pregnant.

Taking care of teeth and gums

The health of your teeth and gums is important during pregnancy. This may seem strange, but germs in your mouth can affect your baby's growth. They can make baby be born too soon. You can also pass germs to the baby after she is born.

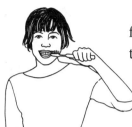

The first step is tooth brushing and flossing. Brush your teeth for two minutes twice a day. Use dental floss once a day. Use a soft toothbrush and floss gently if your gums bleed. And don't eat sugary foods.

Have a checkup by a dentist early in pregnancy. If you don't have a dentist, ask your health care provider who to go to. Make sure to tell the dentist that you are pregnant. Dental care is usually safe during this time.

"I had no idea that my bleeding gums were dangerous for my baby! I'm so glad I went in when I did."

See a dentist right away if you have:

- ◆ red or swollen gums
- ◆ gums that bleed easily
- ◆ bad breath that doesn't go away
- ◆ sores or lumps in your mouth
- ◆ a tooth that hurts or is loose

Don't wait! Work with your dentist to get your mouth healthy quickly.

Hidden dangers around you

The world around you affects your health and the baby's. There can be toxins or germs in the air, water, food, and things you touch. Some are very dangerous during pregnancy.

Simple things like washing your hands often will help limit risk. Take off your shoes in the house and clean your floors often. Use a water filter and open windows for fresh air.

Toxic, poisonous chemicals

Many chemicals can cause health problems for you and baby. There are chemicals hiding in lots of things. Some chemicals have a strong smell. Others give no signs, so you can't tell they're there.

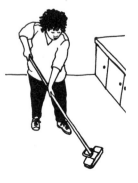

- ◆ Cleaning products—try using natural cleaners instead of harsh chemicals or bleach.
- ◆ Plastics—use plastic food containers and bottles that are not made with BPA. Cloudy plastic is usually safer than clear plastic.

- Fumes—open windows and turn on fans to get rid of bad smells. If you paint or get new carpet, let the house air out. Put new furniture or baby gear in the fresh air for a while before using them.

- Pests—avoid using bug spray or other poisons in or around your home.

- Body care—use soaps, lotions, and sunscreens that are low in chemicals and fragrances.

- Liquid nicotine for e-cigarettes— keep cigarette and refills locked up and away.

Lead in air, water, or inside your home

Lead (led) is a dangerous poison. Eating or breathing even a very small amount can cause miscarriage. It can lead to serious brain damage to unborn babies and small children. It's found in the air, water, and dirt. It is in some paints, plastic, and metal. Some dishes, jewelry, makeup, and even toys have lead in them too.

Lead may be a problem for you if: (check all that apply to you)

____ Your home was built before 1978.

____ You plan to remodel or paint while you're pregnant.

____ Your home has old metal pipes.

____ You or someone in your home works with lead. Some risky jobs are painting, plumbing, construction, car repair, or work with batteries.

Protecting yourself and your family from lead poisoning

Paint on walls and furniture

Old paint is the most common place to find lead in the home. Peeling or cracking paint on walls or outside the house can flake off. Old paint on furniture is very dangerous if kids chew on it.

- If old paint isn't peeling, leave it alone. You can paint over it. But, don't sand, scrape, or burn it first. That would put lead into the air and dust.

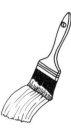

Beware of old paint on furniture or walls. It may have lead in it.

♦ If you have peeling or chipped paint, get it fixed up by a painter. Stay out of the house while they clean up the lead and repaint.

Dirt outside and inside

♦ Take off shoes when you come into the house.

♦ Wash hands well after being outside, before eating, and before sleeping. If you have been gardening or cleaning, use a nail brush. Make sure kids wash hands often, too.

♦ Wet-mop or vacuum floors often to get rid of dust.

Lead in drinking water

♦ Run the water for a few minutes in the morning before using it.

♦ Use only cold tap water for cooking and making coffee or tea. Hot water can pick up lead from old pipes.

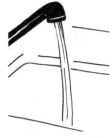

Use cold water for cooking.

Testing for lead

If you are worried about lead, call your health department to learn more. Ask how to test your dirt, paint, or water.

Get rid of lead in your house before baby is born. Babies and young kids crawl around. They often put their fingers or other things in their mouths. (Many kids are tested for lead at their one-year checkup.)

Mercury you might touch or eat

Mercury is very poisonous. If it gets into your body, it can hurt you and your baby. Baby's brain, spine, lungs, and other organs could be seriously harmed.

Mercury is in old glass thermometers and lightbulbs. If one of these breaks, have someone else clean it up and throw it away. Mercury may also be in batteries and old clocks.

Some kinds of fish also have a lot of mercury in them. Fish is good for you while you're pregnant. But, some kinds are better than others. And you don't want to eat too much. Learn more about eating fish safely in Chapter 4.

Germs carried by cats, other pets, and rodents

Cat poop has germs in it that can cause birth defects in an unborn baby even if you don't feel sick. Mice and other small rodents can also carry germs that are dangerous to baby.

Even if the pets seem fine, it's not worth the risk. If you can, have someone clean up after them while you're pregnant. If you must clean up litter yourself, wear gloves. Wash your hands well afterwards.

Heat in hot tubs and saunas

Getting too hot is not good for your baby. It is best not to use a hot tub or sauna while you are pregnant. Stick to warm baths and showers.

Risks of your job

Some problems in pregnancy can be made worse by your work. Even a job where you sit all day can cause swelling and stiffness. Something simple like taking breaks to stretch or walk a few times a day can help.

Are there dangers in your job?

Working around heat, toxins, or machinery can be very dangerous. So can heavy lifting, pulling, or fall hazards. Even caring for others can be risky if there are x-rays, diapers, or other body fluids involved.

Do any of these things sound like your job? If so, talk to your provider. Try to limit how much you are around these things. Ask if there is something else you can do while you're pregnant and breastfeeding.

Is your job hard on your body?

Do you have to sit or stand all day? Do you work shifts that make it hard to get enough sleep? Do you have to lift and carry heavy things? Are you required to work extra-long hours?

Try these things to feel better on the job

- Wear flat shoes and support hose*.
- Do exercises like the pelvic tilt (page 21) to strengthen your back and belly.
- Ask for breaks to walk around or put your feet up.

*Support hose: Snug elastic stockings or socks that calm or lessen swelling and help prevent varicose veins.

If you are having serious health problems, ask your boss if you can do work that's less hard while you are pregnant. If this doesn't work, you may be able to get a leave of absence or go on disability.

Learning to relax more, worry less

How you think and feel affects your body. Keeping your mind free of stress helps you stay healthy. You can learn ways to relax. This will help you find your own way to cope with any difficulties of pregnancy.

What do you think would help you relax?

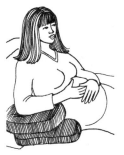

Relax and feel your baby moving, starting in the fourth or fifth month.

____ Practice deep breathing. Close your eyes and relax your face. Breathe in as you count slowly to four, then pause. Breathe out as you count slowly to five. Do this 10 times.

____ Take a nap or spend some time reading.

____ Rest your hand on your belly and feel your baby moving.

____ Learn to knit or sew so you can make a baby blanket.

____ Watch movies that make you laugh a lot.

____ Take a walk in a park with your partner.

____ Have a cup of tea with a good friend.

____ Ask your partner to give you a shoulder rub. Gentle touch can be very soothing.

____ What else helps you relax?

_____

_____

_____

How other people can help you

If something is wrong, tell your partner how you are feeling. That is the only way he or she can know what you are worried about.

Be sure to also tell your doctor or midwife about any problems. Maybe you feel stressed by changes in your job, a move to a new town, or family problems. Your provider can give you better care if he knows what is going on.

Remember: Both you and your partner feel stress at this time. You both will need extra hugs and time to relax, too. You are in this together.

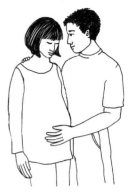

Telling people what you need

We all are part of larger groups. Family, friends, coworkers, and neighbors can help in many ways. If your family is not close, you can make your own with close friends.

You may know that all these people care. But they may not know what they can do to help you. Find ways to tell them what would help you, like this:

- "I'm very tired. Could you please hold my baby, so I can take a nap?"
- "Let's watch a funny movie tonight, not an action film."
- "Please help with the laundry. My back hurts."

Tips for partners

- Go with your partner to her checkups when you can.
- Learn about what she is going through. Read this book. Ask her questions.

- Start healthy habits with your partner. Try cooking new, healthy foods together. Get exercise and relax together.
- Stay healthy. Get your flu shot each fall or winter. Make sure you have had your pertussis (whooping cough) shot (Tdap). Ask your provider about other vaccines you may need.
- Stop your own habits that are not good for baby. It could be as simple as washing your hands when you get home. It could be as hard as quitting smoking. These things show you care.
- Do the dirty work. Painting, cleaning, or other work that uses chemicals should not be done by mom. Scoop the poop. She should not clean up after animals or change the cat box.
- Clear the air. Baby breathes what mom breathes. Don't let anyone smoke near her. Gas the car up for her.

Chapter 4

What You Eat, Drink, and Breathe

Almost everything you take into your body can affect your baby's growth and health. Many things you eat, drink, and breathe pass into your baby's blood. Being good to your body is important for both of you.

Some kinds of foods, drinks, and drugs can harm your growing fetus. You are the only one who can make sure your baby is not exposed to these things. It can be hard to change habits. But that can make a big difference to your baby.

Look in this chapter for:

Good Food: Give Baby the Best page 34
  Smart eating for baby and you
  Choosing the healthiest foods
  Be smart about vitamins and minerals
  Too much of a good thing
Food warnings, page 41
Preparing food safely, page 42
Babies in danger, page 44
  Medicines you've been taking
  Alcohol can harm a child for life
  Cigarettes—Bad for baby
  Serious problems from using drugs
Tips for partners, page 49

Good Food: Give Baby the Best

Smart eating for baby and you

Eating well is one of the most important things to do now to be a good parent. Nutritious foods help your body stay strong. They also help your baby's body and brain develop.

Six healthy eating habits

Now is a good time to start eating better for your family's health. Healthy eating habits are good for you for your whole lifetime.

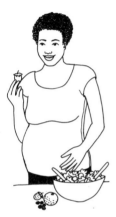

1. Fill half of your plate with colorful vegetables and fruits at meals. Use them as snacks, too.

2. Use whole grain cereals and breads—brown is better than white.

3. Eat meat that is grilled, baked, broiled, or sauteed, not deep fried. Have a variety: fish, chicken, turkey, lean beef. Try tofu or beans instead for some meals.

4. Choose low-fat or non-fat (skim) milk, yogurt, cottage cheese, and soy milk.

5. Drink lots of water! Have fresh fruit and vegetable juice or smoothies instead of soda pop or shakes.

6. Eat less fat. Use oil instead of hard butter or margerine for cooking and bread. Use small amounts of salad dressing and sauces.

Tips for changing your food habits:

- Buy more fresh foods and colorful veggies and fruits.
- Use a grocery list or meal plan when you shop. Keep some healthy foods in the kitchen and your bag at all times.
- Try a new healthy food each week.
- Keep eating healthy foods for your baby. These foods might be new to you, but you may start to like them.
- Remember that exercise goes along with healthy eating.

Nutrients* your body needs

*Nutrients:
Vitamins, minerals, and other things in food that people need to be healthy.

1. **Protein**—for growth of muscles, organs, and cells.
2. **Carbohydrates**—for energy.
3. **Fats**—for energy and cell growth.
4. **Vitamins**—for making the organs, muscles, nerves, and other parts of your body work right.
5. **Minerals**—for healthy growth of bones, teeth, and blood.
6. **Fiber**—for better digestion of foods and prevention of certain diseases.
7. **Water**—for normal working of the entire body. All parts of your body need a lot of water.

If you are under age 18, you need extra protein and foods with calcium, like cheese and milk. This is because your own body is still growing. These foods build your bones and muscles as well as your baby's body.

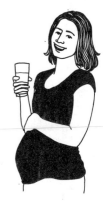

Choosing the healthiest foods

Most people eat too much fat, sugar, and salt in processed foods, fast foods, and snack foods. Learn to make healthy choices. Enjoy the taste of whole grain breads and fresh vegetables. You will be healthier and you often will save money, too.

Here are some of the kinds of foods that give you the most and best nutrients. Try to eat a wide variety of foods, not just your favorites. These foods are best for everyone, not just during pregnancy.

"When I shop for food, I try to get many kinds of food in my cart. Then my meals aren't boring."

Kinds of foods, number of servings each day

◆ **Vegetables** (3 cups)
Broccoli, squash, sweet potatoes, carrots, spinach, collard greens, and bok choy—dark green or bright colored vegetables are best.

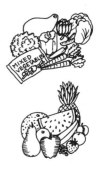

◆ **Fruits** (2 to 3 cups)
Oranges, papaya, apples, melons, blueberries, prunes, and raisins—bright colored fruits are best.

◆ **Whole grains (breads, cereal, crackers, tortillas, pita)**
(6 to 8 small servings), Wheat, oats, rye, cornmeal (masa), rice. Eat a variety each day, not just one kind.

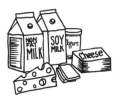

- **Dairy and other calcium-rich foods** (3 cups)
  Non-fat or low-fat milk, hard cheese, cottage cheese, and yogurt. Also, soy milk, most tofu, vegetables, and fish have calcium (see page 40). Read labels on rice or nut milks to check if they have calcium in them.

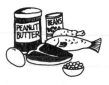

- **Protein foods** (5 to 6 small servings)
  Fish, chicken, turkey, extra-lean beef (10% or less fat), and eggs. Beans, nuts, seeds, peanut butter, lentils, black-eyed peas, cow's milk or soy milk, and tofu. (Avoid some fish, see page 42.)

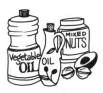

- **Oils** (small amounts)—not hard fats
  Oil from plants like olives, avocado, walnuts, corn, safflower, canola, sesame seeds, or peanuts. (Use in cooking, in salad dressings, and with bread.)

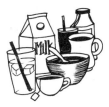

- **Water and other liquids** (8 to10 tall glasses)
  Water is best for you and baby. Milk, fruit or vegetable juice (100 percent juice), and soup are also good. A little bit of coffee and tea is okay, too. (Avoid regular or diet sodas, energy drinks, and sugary juice drinks.)

- **Treats** (have only a little bit now and then)
  Sweets, sodas, white breads, pasta, white potatoes, butter and lard, and processed meats like salami and hot dogs.

How does healthy food fill my plate?

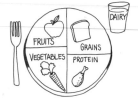

Make sure fruits and veggies fill half your dinner plate.

Healthy serving sizes are smaller than most people think. Eating enough food—but not too much—will help keep your body and your baby healthy.

At first, measure foods when you put them on your plate. That will help you learn how much is too much. See how much space each kind of food should take up on your plate (picture, left).

Vegetarian, vegan, or special diets

You can be very healthy eating a vegetarian or vegan diet. But, you must be careful to get enough protein and some other nutrients. Tell your provider if you eat one of these diets. You may need to take some supplements.

If you don't eat meat, you must make sure you get enough protein, iron, and vitamins B12 and D. Eggs, cheese, and a variety of beans, tofu, and nuts give you protein. Eating lots of vegetables and fruits give you vitamins. But if you fill up on starches like pasta and potatoes you will not get enough nutrients.

If you don't eat milk or egg products, you need to be extra careful to get enough of protein, calcium, B12, and iron. You may need to take B12 and iron pills to get enough of those nutrients.

With all special diets, be sure to talk to your health care provider about the extra good foods you need now. Bring your prenatal vitamins to your next checkup. Ask if there are other vitamins you should take.

What about organic foods?

Organic food may or may not give you more nutrients. But we know organic foods are healthier in many ways. They:

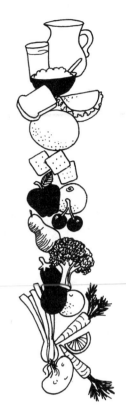

- ◆ are not grown with pesticides (poisons)
- ◆ have no artificial things added, like colors and MSG
- ◆ are grown in ways that are healthy for the earth

Organic foods can be pricey. But many grocery stores and discount stores carry them for less.

Fresh organic foods are not treated with chemicals to make them last longer. This means some may not last as long in your fridge as other foods.

Eating out—Choosing wisely

Going out to eat is great when you're too tired to cook or want to treat yourself. It's also a good way to make some time to talk with your partner. But, choose where you go carefully. Can you get healthy kinds of food there? To keep up your healthy eating habits, make sure to think before you order.

Try to avoid fast food and fried foods. They're high in fat and sodium, and often low in nutrients. If you are in a hurry, try a market that has a soup and salad bar or a deli with fresh foods. Or, order food to go from a restaurant you like.

A restaurant may have some healthy meals, but you still need to be careful. These foods can also be full of fat, salt, and sugar that you and baby don't need. Look for places that serve healthy meals. Don't eat too much. Take home what you can't finish.

Super-sized burgers and sodas aren't really good deals. They're bad for your health.

Tips for Healthy Restaurant Eating

◆ Have a salad with lots of vegetables, beans, and nuts, not just lettuce.

◆ Get salad dressing "on the side" and just use a little bit.

◆ Look for meat that is broiled or baked—not fried or covered with thick sauce or gravy.

◆ Ask for a side of cole slaw instead of fries, if possible.

◆ Have fresh fruit for dessert or just a cup of tea.

◆ Drink water or milk—not soda pop or juice.

◆ Share one large dinner and dessert with a friend or your partner. Or take half of it home for lunch the next day.

Learn to read food labels

Packaged foods have labels to tell you what's in them. The label lists the amounts of protein, fat, salt, calcium, and other things. Check the serving size to know how much to have.

Learn about WIC

The **Women, Infants, and Children Program** ("WIC") is a nutrition program for women who are pregnant, have recently given birth, or are breastfeeding. It also is for babies and kids.

WIC is found in many public health clinics, hospitals, community centers, schools, and housing centers. But it is not just for very low-income families. Once signed up, you can get checks to buy healthy foods. You can also get help with breastfeeding and learn about prenatal care and baby care. WIC staff will help you find other resources in your area.

If your provider does not know how to contact WIC, go to the national WIC website (in Chapter 17) for your state or tribal WIC phone number.

Be smart about vitamins and minerals

While you are pregnant, it is very important to get enough of the right vitamins and minerals. Even a healthy diet may not give you all of every nutrient you need.

Prenatal vitamins

Taking vitamins doesn't replace eating healthy foods. But, it's very hard to get all the vitamins you need from your food. You can be sure you are getting enough by taking prenatal vitamins every day.

Choose a prenatal vitamin that has 100% (percent) of vitamins and minerals you need. Check the label. It is important not to get too many vitamins daily, so don't take other supplements unless your provider tells you to. Most women need extra calcium. Some need DHA, iodine, or iron.

If you don't like to take big pills, you can try capsules instead or cut your pills in half. Be sure to take both pieces in one day. There are also prenatal vitamin gummies or powders that you mix in water. If your vitamin makes you feel sick, try taking it before bed with a snack or try a different brand.

Iron

Iron is in most prenatal vitamins. It's a very important mineral during pregnancy. It's hard to get enough iron from the foods you eat.

Some women worry that iron may make them constipated. But don't skip the iron, it's too important. Here are other ways to prevent constipation:

- ◆ Eat high-fiber foods such as whole grains, bran cereal, and fruits like prunes (dried plums) every day.
- ◆ Drink plenty of water.
- ◆ Ask your provider if you need a fiber pill or drink.

Folic acid

One of the most important vitamins during pregnancy is folate. (It is also called folic acid.) In the first few weeks, it helps prevent very serious defects in the baby's spinal cord and brain. It continues to be important for your baby's growth all during pregnancy. You should have at least 600 to 800 mcg while you're pregnant.

Most prenatal vitamins have at least 600 mcg of folic acid. You can also get some from eating foods like dark green, leafy vegetables, orange juice, dry cereals, breads, and pasta.

Getting enough calcium

While you are pregnant, you need plenty of calcium. Calcium makes your baby's bones and teeth strong. It also keeps your bones strong.

Cow's milk has much more calcium than most foods. But some people find that milk gives them gas, cramps, and diarrhea*. This is called "lactose intolerance." It is very common among people who are African-American, Hispanic, Asian-American, and Native-American. Tell your provider if cow's milk makes you feel sick.

*Diarrhea:
(Die-a-ree-a): Bowel movements that come more often than normal and are very soft and watery.

If you have lactose intolerance, you may be able to eat some foods made from milk. Try yogurt with live cultures, or hard cheese like cheddar or Swiss. You may find "low lactose" milk and pudding easier to eat. Your health care provider may suggest Lactaid or calcium tablets, such as Tums.

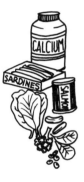

Some other foods also give you calcium, but you need to eat a lot of them to get enough. These are:

- collard greens, kale, cabbage, radishes, bok choy, parsnips, broccoli
- orange juice with calcium added
- fresh or canned salmon or sardines
- some kinds of tofu (check the label)
- corn tortillas made with lime
- black-eyed peas, beans, sesame seeds, almonds, and peanuts
- blackstrap molasses

Iodine

Iodine is needed by pregnant and breastfeeding women to help with baby's development. Use iodized table salt, and eat seafood (cod, seaweed, etc.), milk, and yogurt. Many people don't get enough in their diet or from prenatal vitamins. Ask your provider about taking iodine pills.

Omega-3 fatty acids and DHA

This is important for your baby's development. Your prenatal vitamin may have this. You also can get it from fatty fish (salmon, sardines) or fish oil (cod liver oil), nuts (walnuts) or flax seed oil, or cooking oils (canola, olive). Some foods have it added (fortified orange juice, milk).

Too much of a good thing
Vitamin A

Vitamin A is very important for health, but too much may cause birth defects. You'll get enough in a prenatal vitamin (no more than 5,000 IU) and from eating meats, eggs, and colorful fruits and vegetables. Don't take extra vitamin A or eat liver. Liver has too much vitamin A to eat during pregnancy.

Caffeine

Caffeine speeds up your heart, making you feel more awake. A little bit of caffeine is okay for healthy pregnant women. But, if it makes you jumpy, baby will feel that way, too. Too much caffeine may increase the risk of miscarriage. It also limits how many nutrients you get from food.

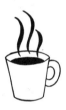

Coffee and tea have caffeine. 1 to 2 small cups of coffee or tea per day (200 mg) is usually safe. Most soda pop and even chocolate have some caffeine. Many cold medicines, headache drugs, and diet pills also have caffeine. Ask your provider or pharmacist before taking any medicines.

Don't drink energy drinks or take any herbs that claim to give you energy or keep you awake. Read labels on sports drinks to make sure they don't have caffeine.

Food warnings
Very salty foods

Everyone needs a little salt every day, but too much is not healthy. Pregnant women with no blood pressure problems can have some salty foods safely. Ask your provider how much to limit your salt.

Salt is in lots of foods that don't taste salty. Vegetable juices, bottled water, sports drinks, and some milk products have it. Some foods, like chips, pickles, fast foods, and pre-made foods, have much more salt than is healthy for anyone.

Some products are now made with less salt than others. Look for the amount of sodium on labels.

Things that aren't really food

Some people want to eat (crave) things that are not food. It may be dirt, clay, ice, laundry starch, or something else. This is called pica.

If you crave things that aren't food, tell your provider. Pica can make you very sick or may be a sign of a health problem. These things do not give you the nutrition you and your baby need.

Food supplements

Dietary food supplements are vitamins, minerals, herbs, enyzmes, and other things. They are labeled as healthy. But, they may or may not be good for you while you are pregnant. Ask your provider before using them. It is better to get your nutrients from real foods—and from your prenatal vitamin.

Mercury in fish

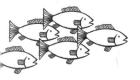

Some kinds of fish are very healthy to eat during pregnancy. You need to choose wisely. Some fish have a lot of mercury in them. Mercury is toxic to unborn babies and young kids. Limit yourself to no more than 12 ounces of healthy fish each week.

Fish to avoid

"I really miss my sushi, but better safe than sorry."

- ◆ Any shark, swordfish, king mackerel, or tilefish.
- ◆ Fish caught in rivers, lakes, and some ocean areas by family or friends. Fish from some waters have different levels of safety. Ask at your local health department before eating.

Kinds of fish OK to eat

- ◆ Shrimp, frozen "fish sticks," sardines, salmon, cod, pollock, tilapia, catfish, or canned light tuna.

Preparing food safely

People often get sick from food that isn't clean, or has gone bad. This can happen if it is stored poorly or kept too long.

Cooking and storing food wisely

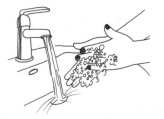

- ◆ Wash your hands well before and after touching food.
- ◆ Cook all meats, poultry, fish, eggs, or shellfish (clams and oysters) well.
- ◆ Eat prepared foods very soon after making or buying them. This means foods like roast chicken, salads, pizza, and sandwiches.

- Keep your refrigerator cold, under 40 degrees.
- Use leftovers soon, within a few days.

Using raw foods safely

- Keep raw meat away from other foods. Don't cut fruits and vegetables on the same board with raw meat.
- After handling raw meat, wash your hands with soap and hot water. Scrub the cutting board, knives, and counters well.
- Wash fruits and vegetables before eating them.

"I love having leftovers. I write the date on a piece of tape and put it on the container. Then it's easy to throw out food if I keep it too long."

Listeria—Serious poison in some unclean foods

Listeria germs cause a bad illness for anyone, especially pregnant women. The germs are in some unclean foods or drinks. They also are found in foods that are not cooked enough.

Listeriosis, the disease, can cause miscarriage, stillbirth, and preterm labor. A baby could be born very small. He could have a deadly infection when he's born.

How to avoid this poison:

- Wash all produce well before cutting, cooking, or eating.
- Cook all meats, poultry, and fish well. Canned fish and packaged seafood can be eaten safely.
- Avoid raw fish, like sushi, and other raw meats.
- Eat prepared meats (hotdogs, lunch meats) only if you heat them first. They should be steaming hot.
- Stay away from soft cheeses like feta, Camembert, queso fresco or blanco, or cheese with blue veins. Hard and semi-soft cheese (such as cheddar and mozzarella), cream cheese, and cottage cheese do not carry listeria.
- Avoid raw (unpasteurized) milk, yogurt, and cheese.
- Wash your hands after going to the bathroom or changing diapers.

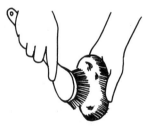

Babies in Danger

Medicines, alcohol, tobacco, and drugs

Some things (substances) you may be taking into your body can cause very serious health problems for you and your baby.

It's important for your health care provider to know about any drugs you may use. Be honest with her. She will help you get treatment. **If you can't stop using any of these things, now is the time to get help.**

Medicines you've been taking

Any medicine you take can get into baby's body through your blood or breastmilk. Now you need to learn if the ones you take are safe for your baby. Be sure to tell your provider about all medicines or other substances you take. These include:

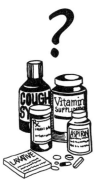

- Medicines prescribed by a doctor before you were pregnant.
- Drugs you can buy over-the-counter, such as aspirin, acetaminophen, vitamins, laxatives, cold medicines, and cough syrup.
- Food supplements, herbs, teas, or drinks.

Alcohol can harm a child for life

If you drink beer, wine, or liquor, the alcohol goes from your blood stream into your baby.

Alcohol can hurt an unborn baby's brain. He could be born too soon or be very small. He could have serious, life-long learning and behavior problems. These are called fetal alcohol spectrum disorders*.

*Fetal alcohol spectrum disorders: Lifelong problems common in kids whose moms drank alcohol while pregnant. These include problems with growth, learning, sleeping, eating, and behaving. The most severe disorder is fetal alcohol syndrome (FAS).

Remember, those first weeks of pregnancy are very important to baby's development. Stop drinking as soon as you think you might be pregnant.

No one knows how much alcohol is safe during pregnancy. This means it is best not to drink at all. Even a little bit can do damage. You don't have to be an alcoholic to have your child affected by alcohol. Alcohol is also passed through breastmilk. So, limit alcohol while you're breastfeeding, too.

Facts about drinking alcohol

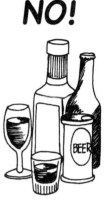

NO!

- ◆ Fetal Alcohol Spectrum Disorders are the most common preventable mental disabilities.

- ◆ A woman's blood absorbs more alcohol from a drink than a man's does. This means the same size drink will affect you more than a man. The alcohol in your blood will affect your baby.

- ◆ There is about the same amount of alcohol in a can of beer, a bottle of wine cooler, a glass of wine, and a shot of hard liquor.

- ◆ "Coolers" and cocktails may not taste strong, but they can have a lot of alcohol in them.

Is it hard to quit drinking?

If you have a hard time not drinking, you may need help. Tell your partner you want to stop. Your provider can help you get counseling. It may be hard to quit, but it will be best for both you and your baby.

Tips to make quitting easier:

- ◆ Stay away from people who are drinking alchohol.

- ◆ If others in your family drink, tell them why you are trying not to drink. Ask them to do other things with you to relax. You could get some exercise or cook a nice dinner together.

- ◆ If you feel like drinking when you are alone, find something else to do. Go see a friend who does not drink, take a walk, or see a movie.

- ◆ Find a support group for people trying to quit.

Your baby is the best reason to quit drinking!

Drinking and driving can hurt too!

Both you and your baby could be hurt if you drink and drive. Riding with a driver who has been drinking is also very dangerous. You and your baby could be seriously hurt or killed in a crash.

Tips for being safe if your driver has been drinking:

- Drive yourself
- Take a cab home
- Ask someone who hasn't been drinking for a ride
- Stay with friends

Be sure to buckle your seat belt whenever you are in a moving vehicle.

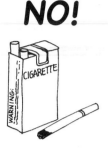

Cigarettes—How bad for baby?

Your baby needs the oxygen you breathe in the air. That oxygen passes into his body through your blood. But, so do the toxins and chemicals you breathe in. When you smoke:

- Nicotine* makes baby's heart beat faster.
- Carbon monoxide* can poison his blood, hurt his brain, and even cause death.
- Smoking can cause miscarriage or stillbirth. Your baby may be born too soon or be very small.
- After birth, babiesof smokers may have more colds, breathing problems, and ear infections than other kids.

*Nicotine:
A chemical in tobacco that is very harmful.

*Carbon monoxide:
A poisonous gas that comes from burning things.

Second-hand smoke

Smoke from other people's cigarettes affects your health. It also reaches your baby in the uterus and can cause harm. If your friends smoke, ask them not to smoke in your home. And stay out of smoky places.

E-cigarettes—Are they safer?

Electronic cigarettes are popular. Just because they're not a lit cigarette doesn't mean they're safe for baby. The liquid that goes in e-cigarettes is made of toxic chemicals like nicotine. The vapor that comes out has those chemicals, too.

E-cigarette vapor isn't as strong as the smoke from a plain cigarette. But it is still not safe for pregnant women or babies and kids. Beware, toddlers and older kids can get into them. Just a drop or two of liquid nicotine is very poisonous for children.

Quitting smoking

This is one of the most important things you can do for your baby's health. Even if you quit in the middle of pregnancy, you are helping your baby.

Ask your provider for help quitting. Talk to him about using a nicotine patch or gum. Also ask your partner and friends to support you while you quit.

Here are some questions to answer:

◆ Why do I want to stop? (ideas: "for my baby's health," or "it's too expensive."):

_____

_____

◆ What can I do when I feel like having a cigarette? (ideas: "have a mint after eating" or "not hang out with people who smoke."):

_____

_____

◆ How much could I save every week by not buying cigarettes?

Do the math. See how much smoking costs you!

$$\frac{\quad\quad\quad\quad}{\text{packs per day}} \times \; 7 \; = \; \frac{\quad\quad\quad\quad}{\text{packs per week}}$$

$$\frac{\quad\quad\quad\quad}{\text{packs per week}} \times \frac{\$\quad\quad\quad}{\text{cost of each pack}} = \frac{\$\quad\quad\quad}{\text{cost per week}}$$

◆ What could I do with the money I'll save? Ideas might be: "hire a babysitter so I can go to the movies" or "save for a car seat for my baby."

_____

_____

◆ What could I say if someone starts smoking near me? Ideas: "please go outside to smoke" or "please don't—it might make me start again."

◆ What date in the next two weeks will I promise myself I'll quit? Write down your quit date: _____.

◆ What are some things I'll do on that day? Ideas: "flush all my cigarettes down the toilet" and "tell my friends and family and ask for their help."

_____

_____

The day you quit

Get rid of all cigarettes and ashtrays in your home, car, and at work. Tell all your friends you have quit and ask for their help.

Take good care of yourself by taking a long walk or going out with non-smoking friends. Every time you want a cigarette, distract yourself with gum or a toothpick to chew on. The feeling will last only a few minutes.

You will probably start feeling better in about two or three weeks. But, if you do start again, don't give up! Set a new date.

Serious problems from using drugs

Any drugs can have serious effects on a pregnant woman and her baby. Many drugs pass to the baby through the umbilical cord. After birth, they are in breast milk. Possible problems include miscarriage, low birthweight, and birth defects.

Prescription drugs

Many people get hooked on prescription drugs. These include sleeping pills, pain killers, or stimulants. People use more than is safe, borrow pills from others, or take them with alcohol or other drugs.

Any of these things could harm your baby. If you do this, it is very important to quit. Be sure to tell your provider everything you are using. You can get help.

Marijuana

Marijuana in your body gets into your baby's blood. It can affect baby's brain and growth. So it is wise to quit using it during pregnancy and breastfeeding. Even a father's use of pot can affect baby.

If you use marijuana for a medical reason, talk with your doctor or nurse about ways to avoid using it now.

Stronger illegal drugs

Drugs like cocaine, heroin, PCP, methamphetamine, and others, are extremely dangerous for unborn babies. When a pregnant woman gets high, her baby does, too. What might make you feel good for a short time may do life-long harm to your child.

Using these drugs even a few times can hurt an unborn child. If you have a drug habit, now is the time to get help and quit. It may not be easy, but having a healthy baby is worth it!

Drugs can cause

- Miscarriage or stillbirth
- Heavy bleeding late in pregnancy
- Preterm birth or low birthweight, which can cause other problems
- A baby born addicted who must go through the pain of withdrawal
- A child who has lifelong trouble learning or behaving

The sooner you can stop smoking, drinking, or taking drugs, the better for both of you. It's hard, but you can do it!

Tips for partners

- Eat healthy foods with mom. Help her shop and cook. Bring her food if she's too tired.
- Fill her water bottle for her.
- Remind her to take her prenatal vitamins every day.
- Help her stop smoking, drinking, or doing drugs. Get these things out of the house. Don't smoke, drink, or use drugs around her.
- Do all these things for yourself, too. It's good for baby to have two healthy parents.

Health Care for You and Baby

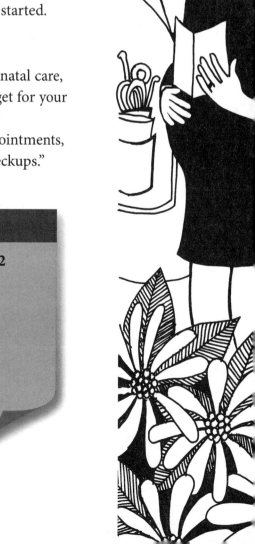

It's important to have a prenatal health checkup at least once a month. Even if you're feeling great, these checkups are one key to staying healthy. These visits to your health care provider help find and treat problems early. Some problems you may not even know you have. Checkups also give you time to ask questions.

You may be able to use the doctor you already go to. If not, you will need to choose a prenatal care provider and a place to give birth. Your choices depend on what kind of care you want before and during birth. The health insurance you have may limit your choices. This chapter will help you get started.

Words about your care

Some words you will hear are maternity care, prenatal care, and obstetrical care. They all mean the care you get for your pregnancy. We will use the words "prenatal care."

Words for visits to your provider include appointments, visits, and checkups. We will use "visits" and "checkups."

Chapter 5

Look in this chapter for:

Choices in prenatal care and birth, page 52

    A place to give birth

    A health care provider

    Prenatal visits—what to expect

Plan ahead: care for baby, page 59

    Choosing your baby's provider

Tips for partners, page 60

Some words used for the birth of a baby are birth, childbirth, or labor and delivery. Usually we will use "birth." Your care after birth is usually called postpartum care.

Choices in prenatal care and birth

The place you give birth, the kind of care you want, and the provider go together. These are very personal choices. So take some time to decide. You want to be comfortable with your provider.

Know what your insurance pays for

Start by talking to your insurance company, employee benefits office, or health clinic. Find out:

- What kinds of prenatal and birth care does your plan pay for?
- How much will you have to pay yourself?
- What options do you have?

The answers to these questions will help you know how much choice you have for place and provider.

If you don't have health insurance now, call or visit your local public health clinic. You may be able to sign up for Medicaid. There also are community health centers that offer low-cost care.

Learn enough to make a good choice

To make these choices, it helps to know what happens during birth. Reading Chapters 6 and 10 will give you a good start. (Use the Glossary in Chapter 17 to find the meanings of words you don't know.)

If you think you want to change providers, you can. But it's easier not to have to change.

Some women choose their doctor or midwife first. Whoever you choose will work at a specific medical center or clinic. He or she will have preferences for the types of delivery they do.

Other women feel strongly about where and how they give birth. They want to choose a birth place first and then find a provider who delivers there.

If you're not sure where to go for care, call:

- your insurance plan
- local public health office

- community clinic
- nearby hospital

Choosing a place to give birth

Different kinds of birth places are good for different reasons. (Read more on the next pages.)

- **Hospital**—all services in one place, may have a focus on using medical ways of birth.

- **Birth center in a hospital**—a blend of medical and natural ways of birth, more choices between medical and natural ways of birth.

- **Birth center outside a hospital**—more personal care, easier to use natural ways of birth, for women with problem-free pregnancies.

- **Your home**—most personal and family-centered, easiest to use natural ways of birth, for women with problem-free pregnancies.

"I asked my friends about where they delivered their babies. But I tried to remember that I might want a different kind of birth than they had."

There are a lot of things to think about before choosing where to have your baby. What kind of birth do you want to have?

Ask your friends where they gave birth and what kinds of medical things were done. Ask what they liked or disliked about the provider and place. Did they use any drugs? Could they get up and move when they wanted?

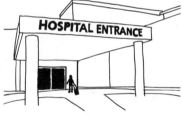

Hospitals and birth centers in hospitals

Hospitals offer all birth services in one place. But not all hospitals have birth care. Look for one with a birth center. A birth center has private rooms set up just for having babies. It looks and feels less like a hospital. Medical machines are covered up and lights are dim. It's quieter than a regular maternity floor.

Things to think about before choosing birth in a hospital:

- You may have many different nurses and doctors or midwives during labor and birth.

- If you want medicine for pain or to help you rest, you can have it.

*Cesarean section:
Surgical birth of a baby.
See Chapter 10, page
156, to learn more.

- If there is trouble during the birth or you need surgery (cesarean section*), it can be done right there.

- You and baby will stay there 1 to 2 days, maybe longer. Nurses will be there to help you recover and teach you how to care for baby. There will be people to help with breastfeeding.

- There are staff to help you with insurance, social services, birth certificates, and other big decisions.

In some hospitals, providers and nurses have a set way of doing things. So, they may expect you to come in, give birth, and recover a certain way. These ways could be simple things like having you wear a hospital gown and lying in bed during labor. Or, they may want to use medical tools early, without waiting for natural ways to work. Things like the use of pain medicine, vaginal exams, and fetal monitors are more likely. A birth center in a hospital may be more open to natural methods.

All of these things might be okay with you, but it's important to think about them now. You may be able to have a natural birth in a hospital, but you may have to push for it.

Private birth centers and birth at home

You may want a more natural birth. You may want to avoid medicines and monitors. You may want to wear your own clothes and move around during labor. You are more likely to be able to have a natural birth outside of the hospital.

A birth center or home birth is only for women who have low-risk pregnancies. You are at "low risk" for problems if you:

- are under 35 years of age,

- are expecting only one baby, and

- have no existing health problems like diabetes.

Of course, sometimes problems start during pregnancy. Your provider may believe a hospital birth is best. It is important to be able to get the care you and baby need if there are problems.

Birth center

A private birth center is like a hospital birth center without the hospital. The rooms are set up like bedrooms. Some may have a kitchen, bathroom, or hot tub, too. Most births are done with midwives. Some doctors deliver at birth centers, too. You go to the birth center when you're in labor, and often leave just a few hours after birth.

Planned home birth

You may want to have your baby at home. This is most often done with a midwife, sometimes with a doctor. You purchase the supplies and your provider comes to you when you're in labor. Basic care after birth is done at home, too.

You may feel most comfortable and private at home. Your kids may be able to be at the birth, too.

Things to know before choosing birth outside a hospital

- Most births do not have problems. Most women do not need drugs or medical help. It helps to have providers who know natural ways to help with birth. But in many areas there are very few doctors or midwives who will deliver in a birth center or at home.

- You will have more choices in labor and birth at home or a birth center. You also will get more help using natural ways to cope with pain.

- Pain medicines **cannot** be used there. If you end up needing them, you must go to the hospital.

- When problems happen, they can happen fast. It's important that your midwife have a trusted doctor to call if there are problems. It could be for advice or to send you to the hospital for care.

- Birth centers often have you go home just a few hours after the baby is born. After a home birth, you won't have to go anywhere.

- Make sure the midwife has a doctor that she would call in case of problems.

- Think ahead. You and your partner probably will both be exhausted. At home there will be no nurse, midwife, or doctor nearby. You may need care yourself. Starting to breastfeed and care for your newborn may give you lots of questions.

- Be sure you know an expert to call if you need help. Also, have an experienced family member or friend, or a doula, to care for and encourage you.

- Though the cost of a birth center is far less than a hospital birth, it is not always covered by insurance.

In the unlikely case of an emergency, think about:

- What hospital would your midwife send you to? How far away is it? To be safe, you should be able to get there in less than 20 minutes.

- If you need to move to a hospital, it can be hard. You would likely have to call 9-1-1 and ride in an ambulance.

Choosing your health care provider

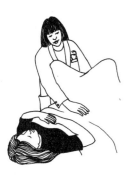

Every woman needs a prenatal provider who is well trained and has delivered lots of babies. You also want someone you trust to give you the best care. This person will be very important to you for the next seven or eight months. Get a list of providers from your health plan.

These are the kinds of health care providers who give prenatal and birth care:

Obstetrician (OB): A medical doctor (MD) with special training in pregnancy and childbirth. An OB (also called an "OB-GYN") can do cesarean surgery.

Midwife: A certified nurse midwife (CNM) is a nurse with special training to deliver babies. A certified professional midwife (CPM) or licensed midwife (LM) is trained as a midwife and is not also a nurse. Use only a midwife who is certified or licensed.

Many midwives work in hospitals and in birth centers. Some do home births. None do cesareans.

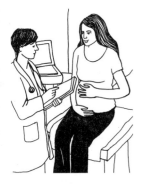

Family practice doctor: A medical doctor (MD) who cares for people of all ages. Some family doctors deliver babies but many don't. They can care for your other medical needs and your baby after birth.

Osteopath (DO): Doctors who have osteopathic training. Some may deliver babies. Some are also midwives, and can give prenatal and birth care. They can also care for you and your baby after birth.

Note: In this book, we will use the word "midwife" for all kinds of professional midwives. We will use "doctor" to mean an OB, a family practice MD, or a DO.

The best provider for you

Try to meet a few health care providers before choosing one. A short "meet and greet" visit should be free. It gives you a chance to get to know these people and to ask questions.

Some of the most important things to ask are about late pregnancy and birth. Learn about these things in Chapters 9 and 10 before you meet providers.

Things to know before choosing

If there is something you feel strongly about, ask about it now. You want a provider who is right for you. Ask these questions.

- *What training have you had in labor and delivery? Are you certified? How many babies have your delivered?*

- *Are there other doctors or midwives who help care for your patients? Will I get to meet them?*

- *Who can I call nights or weekends if I have a question or an emergency?*

- *Do you help women to deliver in the position (sitting, squatting, in tub) that they feel is best?*

- *How do you help mothers handle pain without drugs? If I need something for pain, what do you use most often?*

- *Do you try to avoid episiotomies*?*

- *Do you like a woman to have a birth partner during labor and birth?*

- *What do you usually do if mom's due date passes?*

- *Do you support breastfeeding right after birth?*

"I looked on the Internet at sites that rate doctors. But I wasn't sure that the ratings were true. So I didn't really use them. I trusted my own gut feeling."

*Episiotomy:
A cut made in the skin around the vagina to widen the opening. This can make it easier for the baby to be born.

Questions about cesarean section surgery:

- *When do you recommend a c-section?*
- *What ways do you help women avoid c-sections?*
- *Do you help a woman try vaginal delivery if she has had a c-section before?*

Making your choice

Pick a provider you like and are comfortable with. Make sure he or she respects what you think. Choose one who:

- ☐ Is well trained and certified by the state
- ☐ Listens to and respects your birth choices
- ☐ Has an office that is easy to get to and hours that work for you
- ☐ Can answer your questions by phone or email
- ☐ Can speak your language or use a medical interpreter
- ☐ Has easy access if you have a disability or a TTY phone line if you are hard of hearing

Prenatal visits—What to expect

Your provider will want to see you once a month until your 7th month. Starting in your 7th month (week 29 or third trimester), you should have a checkup every two weeks. In your 9th month (week 37), go in once a week. At 40 weeks, you're at your due date. Your provider will want to see you very often from now on.

You will learn more about these checkups in Chapters 7, 8, and 9. Each chapter has pages to keep notes about your checkups.

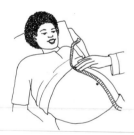

Talking with your provider

Your doctor or midwife will want to give you good care. But you must do your part, too. Your part is to be open and honest. Tell him how you feel and what worries you. Checkups are the best times to talk. But he will want you to call any time something serious comes up.

Write down concerns or questions as you think of them. This will help you remember what to ask at your next visit. There are places to write questions on the checkup pages in Chapters 7, 8, and 9.

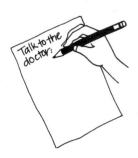

Any time you don't feel well

Be sure to call your doctor or midwife if you feel sick or have pain. See the list of warning signs in Chapter 7.

Things to know before calling your provider (write in the answers here):

How do you feel different from usual?

_____

_____

How long have you been feeling this way?

_____

_____

How have the feelings changed?

_____

_____

Do you have a fever? (Take your temperature and write it down before you call.)

_____

Plan ahead: Care for baby

Your baby will need a lot of checkups, too. So you'll need to pick a provider before he or she is born. You won't have time after you have your baby.

Kinds of providers for babies and children:

Pediatrician: A doctor (MD) with special training in caring for babies and children

Pediatric nurse-practitioner: A nurse with special training in caring for babies and children

Family practice doctor: An MD who cares for people of all ages

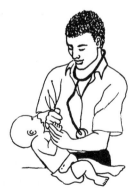

If you already have a family physician, that person could also care for your baby. If not, ask your doctor or midwife to suggest a doctor for baby. Check with your health plan to see which

providers it covers. Ask your friends who their kids see and if they like them. It is best to meet with a few before picking one.

Some questions to ask:

- *Is the clinic or office easy to get to? (You will need to take your baby there often for checkups.) Do the office hours fit your schedule?*
- *Is the provider friendly and easy to talk to? Does he have time to answer questions? Does he have a nurse who can give advice by phone or email when you need it?*
- *Is he easy to reach in an emergency? Who can you call when he is away?*
- *Do his thoughts on baby care match yours? Think about how you feel about things like vaccines, breastfeeding, or sleep.*

Babies and children need to see their provider often even when they are not sick. These are called "well baby visits." Most babies have about seven well baby visits in their first year. See Chapter 15 for more.

How will you pay for your baby's care?

If you have health insurance for your family, the plan will likely cover new babies. You must call the plan before birth to find out how to get your baby covered as he gets older.

If you have no insurance for your baby, call your public health department or community clinic. These places can help you sign up for insurance or Medicaid for yourself and your baby. Ask about the Children's Health Insurance Program (CHIP).

Tips for partners

- Talk to your partner about where she wants to have the baby. Go with her to meet providers.
- Help her find out what is covered by her insurance plan and yours. Ask about having the baby added on.
- Go with her to her checkups. Learn about tests.
- Talk with her about the kind of care you both want for baby. Go with her to meet providers.

Chapter 6

Plan Ahead for Birth and Baby

The basics to learn now

Why is it important for you to think about birth and baby care now? It's best to know something about birth before you choose the kind of medical care you want. Also, it's never too early to start getting ready for your baby's birth. There is a lot to learn.

You'll have important decisions to make before you give birth. In the last months before birth, you will be busy and have less energy than now. You may need time to decide about birth options and breastfeeding. It can take time to get all the things you'll need for baby care. Once you have a baby, you will have very little time for shopping.

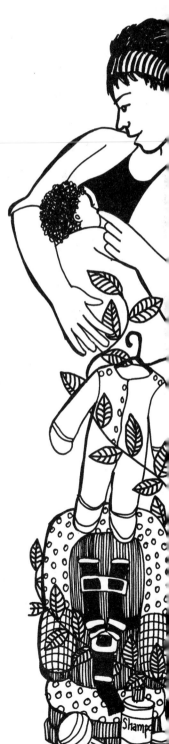

Look in this chapter for:

Preparing for childbirth, page 62

    Learning about birth

    Learning about cesarean section

    Your birth team

Time off from work, page 65

Learning about baby care, page 65

    Feeding your baby

    Why is breastfeeding the best choice

    Is nursing right for you?

    Feeding your baby formula

Things you and your baby will need, page 67

    Choosing the "best" car seat

    Choosing second-hand baby gear

Tips for partners, page 74

Preparing for Childbirth

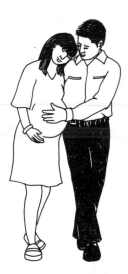

Learning about birth

Birthing a baby is a natural part of life. Having a delivery through your vagina (birth canal) is as normal as having sex. But that doesn't mean it's easy. The more prepared you are, the easier it is.

Most women feel proud and strong after they have a baby. They remember the excitement of birthing their baby more than the pain.

The best ways to get ready for birth:

- **Learn all about the stages of birth.** Learn the basics now by reading Chapter 10. Read about different ways of giving birth. You may need to make some choices that aren't simple. Check out books and websites that you can trust. (See Chapter 17 for resources.)

- **Choose a birth partner.** Having someone with you for support during birth will really help you. It might be your partner, a friend, or a relative. Think of a person who calms you down when you're upset. This person must really want to be in the room during the birth.

- **Take childbirth classes.** Sign up early. Taking a class is very important so you will know what to expect. Many hospitals, clinics, and childbirth groups give classes. Your birth partner should plan to go to these classes with you. They may be quick or last 6 to 8 weeks. You should be done by the end of your 8th month (36 weeks).

"I was really glad my partner stayed with me all the way through delivery. He was a huge help. It meant a lot that he was there to see what I was going through."

Start learning now

Begin with Chapter 10. It covers the basics of natural birth, stage by stage. It also tells about medical things (drugs, surgery) that might be done. Read about natural ways to cope with pain. Find out about epidurals and c-sections. Learn about what options and choices you may have.

Remember that every woman and every birth is different. Also, many things have changed a lot from your mom's day.

"Some of my friends tried to tell me about their deliveries. I had to ask them for helpful stories, not horror stories."

Coping with pain

Giving birth is not going to be comfortable. You can't avoid all the pain, even with drugs. The pain will be easier to cope with if you know what's happening. Knowing how to relax and having a birth partner also helps a lot. Keep in mind that the pain will go away between contractions and almost as soon as your baby is born.

You may hear that it is easiest to have drugs for birth. Learn about the good and bad sides of drugs. Side effects and problems don't happen often, but they can be serious. Labor and birth without drugs is possible for many women. Learn about your options.

Learning about cesarean section

A cesarean section (c-section) is major surgery to take a baby out of the uterus. The mom is given drugs in her spine so she can't feel much below the chest. The doctor makes a cut into the mom's belly and the uterus. Then baby is pulled out of the hole and the mom is stitched back up.

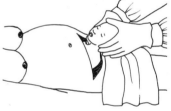

A c-section is necessary if there's an emergency with mom or baby. Some problems can make a vaginal birth too risky. Then a c-section is the safest way to go.

Today, c-sections are often done for less serious reasons. However, medical experts now say it's often not the best option for a healthy mom and baby. There is a higher chance of problems or death from a c-section than a vaginal birth.

A cesarean section is surgery to get baby out fast.

Vaginal birth after cesarean

Most women who have a c-section end up having surgery for later babies, too. But, that's changing. Many moms want to have a vaginal birth next time. This is called vaginal birth after cesarean (VBAC, pronounced "vee-back").

VBAC is usually very safe, but not all providers or hospitals will help a mom do it. If you want to try VBAC, it's best to choose a doctor or midwife who has experience with VBAC.

Your birth team

Nurses and doctors will come and go during your labor. Even a midwife may not stay with you until it is time to push the baby out. It's good to have someone stay with you the whole time to help. This is your birth partner (sometimes called a labor coach).

Your birth partner can help you use the breathing and relaxation methods you learn in childbirth class. He or she can help you remember your goals and wishes, and help you to be as comfortable as possible.

Find someone who can go to classes with you. They may need to take time off from work or away from their family for the birth. You might ask two people, in case one can't be there the whole time.

Is your birth partner a good fit?

Giving birth is very personal. You want to be around people who will be calm, loving, and supportive. Try not to invite anyone who makes you stressed or uncomfortable. This can make labor harder.

Some people may be scared or upset by the idea of being part of a birth. Your partner or the baby's dad may not want to be there. If he or she feels that way, try to understand. Find someone else, maybe a good friend, your mom, or a doula.

How could a doula help you?

*Birth doula:
A person who has trained to help parents during and right after birth.

A birth doula* is someone trained to help families in labor and birth and newborn care. She is there to support the mom by comforting, explaining, and encouraging. She is also there to help any other partners be as useful as possible. A doula can also help the mom understand what the provider says and explain what is going on.

Women who have doulas often have shorter labors and better feelings about their births than those who give birth without doulas. There is less pain medicine use and fewer c-sections. They often have an easier time breastfeeding, and have healthier babies.

Most doulas work privately. Some hospitals have volunteer doulas for women who don't have one. There are also programs in some areas that offer doulas for little or no money to those in need. If you are an immigrant, you may find a doula who is from your culture and speaks your language. Ask your doctor or midwife to help you find one. (See Chapter 17 for more.)

Arrange time off from work

You will need some time off from work after your baby is born (maternity leave). Plan ahead.

Ask for as much maternity leave as you can get. It takes time to recover from birth. The first few months of parenthood can be very tiring. Also, you and your baby need time to get to know each other and bond with each other.

Learning About Baby Care

Learn all you can now. Most moms and babies come home just one or two days after birth. You won't have time or energy for classes once baby's born. There's so much to know about, like breastfeeding, safe sleep, first aid and CPR* for babies, home safety, and car seat use.

There are many ways to learn. Do what works best for you. Include your partner, friends, or anyone who might take care of your baby.

*CPR: Cardio-pulmonary resuscitation. A way to save a life when a person isn't breathing. Infant CPR is very different from CPR for adults.

- ◆ Read Chapters 11 to 15 for the basics. Read the rest of this chapter about the things you can start getting now.

- ◆ Go to new-parent classes at the hospital or birth center.

- ◆ Watch a video on infant care.

- ◆ Spend time with new moms or dads and their babies.

Breastfeeding your baby

One big decision is about breastfeeding (also called nursing). Breastmilk is best for babies. Some families nurse for a few weeks, some nurse for years. Nurse your baby for as long as you can.

It can be hard to decide so early. Take your time to learn about it.

Why is breastfeeding the best choice for most moms and babies?

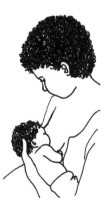

1. Breast milk gives babies exactly what they need until they are at least 6 months old. As baby grows, the milk changes too, so it's always perfect for his needs.

*Antibodies:
Cells made in the body to fight germs. A mom's antibodies get to the baby through breast milk.

2. Only breast milk can protect baby from germs. It gives him antibodies*. He's less likely to have colds, allergies, ear infections, diarrhea, and other problems than babies who are fed formula.

3. Breastfeeding helps you and your baby feel close. This can be especially helpful when you go back to work. Your baby can drink breast milk by bottle while you're gone. He'll still nurse when you are home.

There are lots of great things about breastfeeding. Check out this list of the perks of breastmilk. Mark the ones that help you want to breastfeed.

___ Breast milk is free!

___ It's clean, safe, and ready when you need it. It's the perfect temperature when you nurse him.

___ You can feed your baby when he's hungry, almost anywhere you are.

___ Breast milk in the first few weeks has extra good stuff in it for baby.

___ It has antibodies to help your baby fight germs.

___ Even small breasts can make plenty of milk.

___ Night feedings are faster and easier when nursing.

___ Breastfeeding lets your baby eat just as much as he needs. Breastfed babies are less likely to be overweight as they grow up.

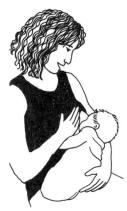

"Formula is so expensive! And what a pain to carry around bottles and nipples, measure the formula and water, mix it up, and heat it. Breastfeeding has been so much easier!"

___ It's a natural thing for your body to do. Even if it takes some time and help, it's an easy way to feed baby for most moms.

___ Moms who breastfeed (or pump their milk) are healthier. Their feelings and their bodies recover from birth faster. Their periods may stay away longer. They're less likely to get cancer, diabetes, and other health problems later in life.

For more on breastfeeding, see Chapter 12.

Breastfeeding and working

You can continue to breastfeed after you go back to work. Many women do this by pumping their breasts while at work. They take the breast milk home so baby can drink it from a bottle.

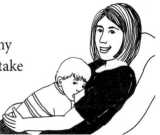

"Is nursing right for me?"

If you are still not sure you want to breastfeed, take some time. Think about why. Is it something you've heard? Have people tried to talk you out of it? Maybe it's just hard to imagine doing it? Remember, breastfeeding is different for everyone. But it can be hard to try a new thing.

Talk with an experienced mom who breastfeeds to learn what it's like.

Think about all the good things about breastfeeding for both your baby and yourself. Talk to people who have enjoyed breastfeeding. Ask them what helped them get started. Ask how it's been to keep breastfeeding for months or years.

The choice is yours. Only you will know what's right for you and your baby. But, you may not know for sure until you try. You **can** do it if you want to.

Feeding your baby formula

Some moms can't breastfeed or choose not to. They may have had too much trouble nursing or felt formula was a better fit for them. See Chapter 12 to learn more on feeding your baby.

Babies who are not breastfed should always drink formula, not plain cow's milk, soy milk, or other kinds of milk. Formula is made to be as much like breast milk as possible. However, it does not have all the nutrients of your milk. It also costs a lot of money.

"My best friend told me, 'When I am nursing, I know I'm doing something no one else can do for my baby. I feel very feminine and beautiful, even if my hair's dirty and I didn't get much sleep last night.'"

Things you and your baby will need

Now's a good time to start thinking about getting clothes, a car seat, and other baby things. It will take time to get all the things your baby needs.

You can get good used clothes and toys from friends, baby gear swaps, and thrift shops. Be careful of second-hand car seats, cribs, and other baby gear. (There is more about second-hand things later in this chapter. Read more about safety in Chapter 14.)

Things for baby

☐ **Diapers:** cloth, disposable, or both. Just get 1 to 2 packages of newborn diapers, since he'll outgrow them fast. You'll need more of the next size up. Cloth diapers can costs less over time, be gentler on baby's skin, and make less trash. But, they take time to wash. They may be hard to use if you don't have your own washing machine and dryer. Disposables are faster and easier, but cost more and make a lot of trash.

*Onesies:
Long shirts that snap at the crotch.

☐ **Warm sleepers with legs, onesies*, socks, a warm hat.** Most babies outgrow the newborn sizes very quickly, unless they're born very small. Get more in sizes 3 to 6 months. A sleep sack can keep baby warm without the risk of blankets in the crib.

*Car seat:
A special seat to keep baby safe in motor vehicles. Also called a "car safety seat" or a "child restraint."

☐ **A car seat*** that fits a new baby. Use it on every ride, starting with the trip home from the hospital. This is the law in every state. It's the best thing you can do to protect your baby's life. (More on car seats later in this chapter and in Chapter 14.)

☐ **A safe place to sleep**, like a crib or bassinet. It must be sturdy, let baby lie flat, and have a firm mattress that fits snugly. You will want a waterproof pad and a few fitted sheets. (More on safe sleep in Chapter 14.)

☐ **Medicine for baby:** Acetaminophen (non-aspirin) baby pain reliever (such as Tylenol) just in case. (Give no ibuprofen to babies less than six months old. Give no aspirin to a child of any age.)

☐ **Thermometer:** Get a plain digital thermometer to check for fever. (See Chapter 15 for more.)

☐ **First aid kit:** Buy or make a first aid kit with bandages, cleaning wipes, and an ice pack for your home. You can get smaller ones for the car and diaper bag.

Things for you

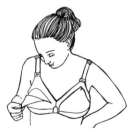

Regular nursing bra with flaps that open.

☐ **Nursing bras.** Start with a stretchy nursing bra or "sleep bra." (These can even help with sore breasts during pregnancy.) After your milk comes in, you might want a regular nursing bra.

These have cups that open in front for breastfeeding. Breast
pads may help when your breasts leak.

☐ **Bottles and nipples:** If you plan to breastfeed, you may need
just a few bottles and nipples for when you pump your breasts.
For formula feeding, you will need some newborn formula
and at least 8 bottles and nipples.

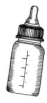

Other useful things

☐ **A nursing pillow:** a curved pillow that fits around your body
on your lap. It helps support baby while nursing.

☐ **A baby tub:** A small plastic bath tub with a sloping back or a
foam cushion can help you bathe baby safely.

☐ **A rocking chair:** Rocking in your arms makes many babies
feel happy and calm.

☐ **A yoga ball:** Bouncing gently on an exercise ball while you
hold her can be very soothing for a new baby.

☐ **A baby carrier:** Use a cloth baby carrier that holds your baby
up high against your chest. It's helpful while doing chores or
shopping. It's also great for a fussy baby. Try it on before buying
and use it right. (See page 225 for carrier safety.)

☐ **A bouncy seat:** A baby seat that rocks or bounces can calm
baby. It is also good to have a safe place to put baby when your
arms need a break. Always use the seat harness and keep baby
where you can see him. This is not a safe place for baby to sleep
for long or be left alone.

☐ **A pacifier:** Sucking can calm a fussy baby. Your breast is best,
but a clean finger or baby's own fingers will work, too. But
save the pacifier for after the first month, after breastfeeding is
going well. Get one made all in one piece.

A one-piece pacifier

☐ **Baby toys:** Rattles, bells, and crinkly things are sounds babies like.
Soft, washable toys are good. Toys shouldn't have small parts (like
buttons or plastic eyes she could chew off.) If a toy fits in a toilet
paper tube, it's too small for baby to play with. He could choke on
it. Avoid toys with small batteries or cords that could get wrapped
around his neck. Remove toys if baby falls asleep.

☐ **Choose colorful things:** Young babies can see bright colors and
black and white shapes best.

$$ Save money:
Bed pillows
work well for nursing.
And a clean sink or a
big dishpan makes a
good tub while baby
is small.

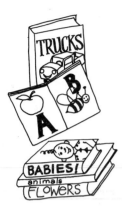

☐ **Books, handouts, and videos:** Collect information on baby care from your clinic, doctor's office, or bookstore. Look on the Internet for more. See Chapter 17 for books and web sites that are helpful and that you can trust.

☐ **Picture books**: It's never too early to start reading short picture books to baby. Pick colorful books with words that rhyme.

Choosing the "best" car seat

Riding in a car is one of the most dangerous times for kids. A car seat does a very good job of protecting your baby or child in a sudden stop or crash. But make sure you use it right.

There is not one "best" car seat for everyone. Try the car seat in your car before you buy it. Make sure it fits and can be tightly fastened. If it can't be installed right, take it back. For more about using car seats, see Chapter 14.

The best car seat for your new baby:

◆ Will fit a small baby by weight and height

◆ Can be used so baby faces the back of the car

◆ Can be buckled tightly in the back seat

◆ Has a harness that's easy to adjust, so you will use it right on every trip

Kinds of car seats for babies

There are two kinds of car seats you could get for your new baby. Both cover a wide range of weights and ages, so read the labels carefully.

1. **A rear-facing car seat** can only be used rear facing. Most babies will outgrow these (be too tall or too heavy) between 8 and 24 months old. This kind:

    ◆ Is easy to carry in and out of the car

    ◆ Often has a base that can stay installed in the car.

    ◆ May be the most useful when baby is small, but he may outgrow it before he is 2 years old. That is when he is old enough to ride forward facing. So you may still have to buy a convertible seat later.

    ◆ May click into a matching stroller

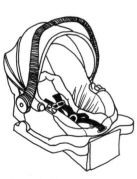

Rear-facing car seat

2. **A convertible car seat** can be used facing the rear for a baby or toddler. When the child gets too big, the seat can be faced forward. Some convertibles may fit your child all the way until grade school. This kind:

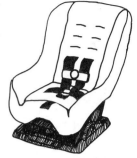

- ◆ Stays secured in the car. You take baby in and out each time you get in and out of the car.

- ◆ Must have a very low shoulder strap setting to fit a new baby well. The more harness settings it has, the longer it will fit your child.

- ◆ Often has higher height and weight limits than a rear-facing only car seat. This means your child can ride rear facing at least 2 to 3 years.

$$ A convertible car seat will give you the best "bang for your buck." It will last the longest.

A more expensive seat is not always safer. All must pass the same tough safety tests. The fit of the car seat in your car and for your baby are most important. There are some great car seats that don't cost a lot and fit new babies well. See Chapter 14 for how to find your local car seat group for help.

If you find it hard to pay for a new car seat, start saving now. Ask your hospital or clinic if they offer low-cost car seats. Find out if your health insurance plan covers car seats. Or, put it on your "wish list" for someone to give as a gift.

Learn how to use the car seat

Get the car seat early. Practice putting a baby doll into the seat. Tighten and loosen the harness. Practice buckling the car seat into your car facing the rear.

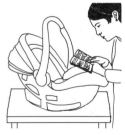

Most people don't use their baby's car seats correctly. Mistakes could put your baby in great danger. Follow the car seat and vehicle instructions. Read Chapter 14 for details about using a car seat correctly.

Read the car seat directions to learn how to adjust the harness and install the seat in your car.

Not every car seat fits well in every car. If the one you have does not fit tightly in your car or you have questions, have it checked before the baby comes. Find a trained Child Passenger Safety Technician in your area (see Chapter 17).

Choosing second-hand baby gear

Buying all new things for your baby is expensive. Getting some kinds of used baby gear costs less and is good for the Earth. You can find some great deals on baby clothes and toys at yard sales and resale shops. They often look as good as new. You can also find deals on bigger baby gear, but you must make sure it's safe.

Beware: some used things can be dangerous, even if they look safe. Especially things that you put your baby in. Used car seats, cribs, baby carriers, playpens, strollers, and play seats can have serious safety problems. For example, the slats on older cribs were further apart, so babies could get their heads stuck and not be able to breathe.

Problems with used car seats

Try to buy a new car seat, if you can. Old car seats are dangerous. Newer car seats are much safer. Even if you don't get a fancy one. See Chapter 14 for more about car seats. When looking at a used car seat, find out:

- **Has the car seat been used in a crash?** Most car seat companies say the seats should not be used after any crash, even a small one. It may have hidden damage you can't see. If you don't know its history, don't use it.

- **Does it have its instructions and all its parts?** It's important to follow the instructions because not all car seats work the same way. You can get new instructions or parts from the company (check their website).

- **How old is it?** Check the "expiration" date on the sticker or the back of the car seat. Many companies say not to use car seats more than 6 years old. A car seat older than 10 years must be thrown away. (Take it apart first, so they can't be found and re-used.)

- **Has the car seat been recalled?** Many recalls are for serious safety hazards. To find out, call the car seat company with the model number and manufacture date or go to *Recalls.gov*. If a used seat doesn't have a sticker with the date and number, there is no way to know it's safe. Don't use it.

Dangers of other used baby gear

Look for the label "JPMA Certified" on any other baby gear you get. Make sure it hasn't been recalled, has all of its parts and instructions, and is in good shape. If you're not sure, don't use it.

Check for baby gear recalls at www.saferproducts.gov

Cribs

Buy a new crib and crib mattress, if you can. There was a big safety update to cribs made after June 2011. If you can't get a new crib, make sure the one you get is safe. Call the company to see if it's been recalled. Make sure the slats (bars) are close enough together that a soda pop can can't go through. It shouldn't have sides that slide down or posts or knobs at the corners.

Playpens or play yards

Don't use a playpen that has been recalled. Make sure the locks on each side work. Get the instructions so you know it's put together right. Playpens with sides that fold down all the way should not be used. (Sides that fold in half and make a "V" are much safer.)

Baby gates

There are gates that bolt into the wall and gates that stay put using pressure. There are gates that open like a door (walk-through) and others that you must step over or take down to get through. Gates for two kinds of openings are:

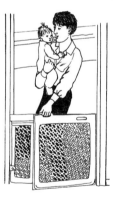

Walk-through gate

- **Doorway gates** can be the pressure or bolt kind. Walk-through gates are less likely to cause falls than the kind you step over. If it's a door you go through often, use a walk-through gate.

- **Stair gates** must be bolted into the wall or railing and must be the walk-through kind. It is too dangerous climb over and risk falling down the stairs.

Look for gates that are smooth on top. Be careful of old folding gates with big diamond-shaped holes. They can strangle a baby.

For product safety and recall resources, see Chapter 17.

Tips for partners

- Learn about birth. Go to classes with mom.
- If you don't think you want to be the birth partner, be honest with her.
- Learn about baby care.
- Take parental leave if you can. It will help you bond with baby. Talk with your boss.
- Support her breastfeeding as long as she can. It may seem strange to you, but it is natural for baby and mom.
- Help choose a car seat. Learn how to install it in the back seat. Go to a car seat check to make sure you've got it right.
- Help get baby's gear ready. Put together the crib. Learn how to use your baby carrier.

Chapter 7

Your 9 Months to Get Ready

The first three months

You have begun a big adventure. Your body and your baby will change a lot in nine months. So take a deep breath.

The nine months are divided into three parts called "trimesters." Each trimester has three months in it. The first trimester is covered in this chapter. The next two chapters are about the second and third trimesters.

The first part of each chapter is about your baby's growth and how your body is changing. The next part covers things you may want or need to know during that trimester.

The last part of each chapter covers your health care visit. There are places to write down questions you want to ask your provider.

In this chapter you will find:

Trimesters, months, and weeks, page 76

Weeks 1 through 12, page 78

 How your baby is growing

 How your body is changing

 Taking care of yourself

Warning signs—Emergency, page 83

Keeping up your healthy habits, page 87

Facts about partner abuse, page 88

Common worries: twins, birth defects, page 89

Warning signs of a miscarriage, 90

Tips for partners, page 93

Month-to-month checkups, page 94

Trimesters, months, and weeks

Many women think about the months of pregnancy. However, your provider may talk about it in weeks. This is because your unborn baby grows so much during each week. There will be about 40 weeks from the start of your last period until your baby's birth.

This is how the weeks and months are divided up:

1st trimester = months 1 to 3 = weeks 1 to 12

2nd trimester = months 4 to 6 = weeks 13 to 27

3rd trimester = months 7 to 9 = weeks 28 to 40

Most women feel different in each trimester. During the first part, you may be uncomfortable as your body gets used to being pregnant. In the second trimester, you will probably feel more comfortable. Pregnancy may seem easier.

In the third trimester, you may have more aches and pains. As your uterus gets really big, it pushes against other organs. Your hips and pelvis get ready for birth. You may wish that baby would come soon. However, the longer she stays inside, the better.

How your body changes as your baby grows

1st trimester   *2nd trimester*   *3rd trimester*

Main things to keep in mind

You've already learned a lot about caring for your body and your baby. Go back and read the tips in Chapters 2 through 6 as often as you need to. These are the biggest things to keep in mind for your whole pregnancy:

☐ Go to all of your prenatal visits.

☐ Learn about pregnancy, birth, postpartum, and baby care from people, books, and websites you trust.

☐ Talk to your partner or your loved ones about how you're feeling. If you feel depressed, tell someone.

☐ Call your doctor, midwife, or nurse if you ever feel that something is wrong in your body.

At prenatal visits, your provider will look at how baby is growing. He'll also check your health. These visits are the best time for you to ask questions. They also help the provider get to know you. You should also get to meet the other doctors or midwives who may care for you when your provider is out.

Your regular checkups will include:

◆ weight

◆ temperature

◆ blood pressure

◆ lungs

◆ breasts

◆ uterus size

◆ baby's heartbeat (starting in the 4th month)

As your pregnancy goes along, your provider will use ultrasound to look at the baby's growth, the placenta, and the uterus. Usually, you and your partner will be able to see the ultrasound screen. You may be able to get a printed picture of the baby. If you want to know if your baby is a boy or girl, he will use ultrasound to find out. If you don't want to know, be sure to tell them before ultrasounds.

Your provider will check your blood type. He will also test your blood and urine for problems you may not feel. These include anemia, diabetes, and infections. If any test is positive, he will run more tests. If there is a problem, he'll tell you how to treat it. If you aren't sure, ask questions.

Things about you could affect your pregnancy

Some people are more likely to have problems in pregnancy. This can be because of your own health history or your ethnicity or race. Ask your provider if there are risks you need to know about.

First Trimester: Months 1, 2, and 3

Weeks 1 through 12

The first three months of pregnancy are very different for everyone. Some don't tell people they're pregnant yet. Some don't look or feel pregnant yet. Others feel it at the very beginning and tell people right away. No matter how you feel in these first months, there are amazing things going on inside of you.

Your baby in your body

Look at the picture on the opposite page (Words in bold below are shown in the picture). Your unborn baby lives in your **uterus** (womb). She is called an **embryo** during the first 8 weeks. After that time, she is a called a **fetus.** (We will use the word "baby" for all stages.) She is curled up in the **amniotic sac** (bag of waters) filled with **fluid (water).**

Her **umbilical cord** is attached to the placenta. The **placenta** is attached to the inside of your uterus. The blood in the placenta and cord carries food and oxygen from you to your baby. It can also carry things that could harm your baby, like alcohol or nicotine. It takes away waste from your baby's blood.

First trimester—How your baby is growing

Your baby in month 1 (1 to 4 weeks after your last period started)

At first, your unborn baby is much too small for you to feel. By the end of month 1, she's almost as big as a grain of rice.

- Her most important organs (lungs, heart, brain, and spinal cord) are forming.
- Her head has little spots that will become her eyes.

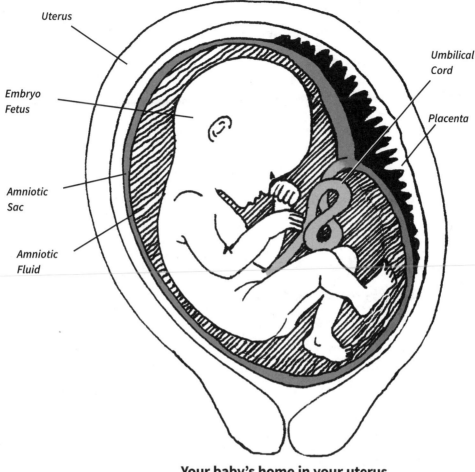

Uterus

Umbilical
Cord

Embryo
Fetus

Placenta

Amniotic
Sac

Amniotic
Fluid

Your baby's home in your uterus

Look back at the pictures of your baby's growth (Chapter 1, page 2, and Chapter 3, page 17). See the amazing changes in just a few weeks.

Month 2 (5 to 8 weeks)

Your baby is starting to look like a person. She has tiny eyes, ears, and a mouth. She will grow to be about one inch (25 mm) long, about the size of a walnut.

- ◆ Her heart is beating by week 5.
- ◆ She now has the beginnings of all the organs and systems that she will have at birth.
- ◆ Her placenta is formed and working.
- ◆ Arms and legs are forming, with tiny fingers and toes.
- ◆ Her brain is growing very fast, so her head is much bigger than her body.

"It is hard to believe that her heart is beating and she already has fingers and toes. I barely feel pregnant yet!"

Month 3 (9 to 12 weeks)

- By the end of month three, your baby will be almost 3 inches (7.5 cm) long.
- She'll weigh about 1 ounce (28 grams).
- Her heart is beating very fast. It's loud enough for your provider to hear.
- Fingers and toes are well formed.
- Her jaws have 20 tiny bumps that will become teeth.
- She can move her arms and legs now. But her kicks are too small to feel.

First trimester—How your body is changing

Your body in month 1 and 2

- About 2 weeks after your period starts, your egg and the sperm come together through sex or fertility help. This is conception, the start of your baby.
- You will have no period about 2 weeks after conception. By now your baby is attached to the wall of your uterus.
- You may start feeling sick to your stomach (nauseous— naws-ee-us) and tired.
- Your breasts will start to feel full and may get sore. Your nipples will start to get darker.
- Your skin may feel dry and you may get more pimples than usual.
- You may get a dark line down the middle of your belly.

Month 3

- You may be starting to gain weight. By the end of this month, you probably will have gained 2 to 5 pounds (1 to 2.25 kg). You may need some bigger clothes soon.
- Your breasts may feel very heavy. This is normal. You may need bigger bras that fit well.
- By the end of this month, you may be able to feel your growing uterus.

- You may get constipated more often than before. Eat plenty of fiber, especially fruit, whole grains and bran. Drink a lot of water, too. Ask your provider before taking any medicine for constipation.

First trimester–Taking care of yourself

Start taking care of yourself right away! Some of your baby's most important growth happens in these first months. Follow the healthy habits in Chapters 2 and 3.

Stay healthy

- Go to your prenatal visits. Learn about pregnancy.
- Eat the healthy foods that you and your baby need. Take your prenatal vitamins every day.
- Get plenty of rest. Take time to sit down, take deep breaths, and relax.
- Get some exercise every day. Walk instead of driving when you can. Take the stairs instead of the elevator at work. Park far from the door when you go shopping.
- Drink lots of water. Skip the sodas and energy drinks. Slices of fruit or cucumber mixed with sparkling water makes a yummy drink.
- Floss and brush your teeth and gums. Go to the dentist and get any problems treated. Tell them you are pregnant.

Stay safe

- Don't use tobacco, alcohol, or drugs. Stay away from places where others are smoking or using. Ask people not to smoke in your car or home.
- Wear your seat belt on every car ride.
- Protect yourself from STDs if you or your partner have sex with other people.
- Ask your provider or a pharmacist before taking any medicines. Tell them you are pregnant.

Feel for the top of your uterus. Push gently on your belly just above your pubic hair and pubic bone. Your uterus will feel round and hard, like an orange.

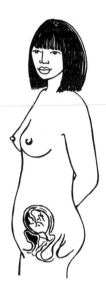

If you don't like drinking plain water, put a little fruit juice into it. Unsweetened sparkling water makes it even more yummy.

Why am I so tired?

In the first few months, you may feel very tired. Growing a baby is hard work for your body! Eating well, exercising, and getting more sleep will give you more energy. Take naps and go to bed a bit earlier than normal. If you want to rest, learn to say "no" to friends who want to go out. Your energy will come back in the next trimester.

What can I do if my stomach is upset?

In the first two or three months, you may feel like throwing up often. You may even vomit daily. This is called "morning sickness" but it can happen at any time of day. It usually stops after the first trimester. Here are some things that may help:

- Eat small meals every two or three hours. Don't wait until you feel really hungry. Bring snacks with you when you go out. Eat a small snack before going to bed.

- Keep some plain crackers next to your bed. Eat a few crackers before getting up in the morning or when you start to feel sick.

- Sip a little fizzy water or ginger ale.

- Eat only the food that you feel hungry for. Don't worry right now if it's not the most nutritious. Eat what you can keep down. You can eat healthy foods when you feel better.

- Stop eating foods that make you feel sick, especially greasy or spicy foods.

After you vomit, rinse your mouth with baking soda mixed with water. Then spit it out. This keeps the acid in vomit from hurting your teeth.

- After you vomit, wait a few hours before eating. Then start with water or weak tea with a little sugar. This gives your body back the liquid it has lost.

- Vitamin pills could upset your stomach if you haven't been eating. Try taking them with food. Or try to take them before you go to bed, so you can sleep through any burps.

Sometimes the smells or sounds around you make you feel sick. Stress, anger, and worry can also make it worse. Talk to your partner, friends, and family. Tell them how you're feeling and how

Warning Signs—Emergency

Learn these warning signs of health problems during pregnancy. Call your health care provider if you think you might have any of them.

- Bleeding from your vagina
- Sudden swelling of your face, hands, feet
- Dizziness
- Trouble seeing
- Bad headaches
- Pain or cramping in your belly
- Pain while urinating (peeing)
- Thoughts of harming yourself or the baby

they can help you. They may not know that their perfume, smelly food, or loud music is making you sick.

If you're vomiting every day, call your provider. Also call if you get dizzy or pass out. They can try to help and make sure your body has enough fluids.

Why do my moods change so much?

In the first three months, your moods are likely to go up and down like a roller coaster. This is very normal. It is from hormones changing in early pregnancy. Most women's moods calm down after month three.

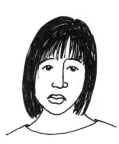

You may have fears or worries about birth or your baby's health. This is normal, too. Sharing your thoughts can help. Learning more may make you less afraid.

- *I'm worried that my baby won't be normal.* Most babies are born healthy. You will have tests during pregnancy to find some of the rare problems a baby might have. Ask your provider about these tests. Meanwhile, do what you can to have a healthy baby.

- *I'm scared of what labor will be like.* A childbirth class will help you know what to expect. You'll also learn ways to cope with pain. You can also read and watch videos about birth. (See Chapter 10 and use resources in Chapter 17.)

◆ ***What if I'm not a good mom?*** It's normal to worry that you might not be the best parent. Remember that everyone has to learn how to be a good parent. You can practice by helping to care for a friend's baby. Talk to other moms about what it's been like for them.

Things to do to help yourself feel better

◆ Learn to cook some new and healthy recipes.

◆ Take a walk every day. Going with a friend can be more fun than going alone. It also gives you time to visit.

◆ Try learning something new, like knitting. You could make a little hat for your baby.

◆ Do something nice for someone, like babysitting for a friend or visiting an elderly neighbor.

◆ Have a girls' night out with your friends. Go to a funny movie.

◆ Ask your partner to rub your neck and shoulders.

Talking about feelings can help

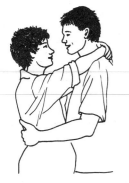

If you are feeling blue, tell someone who cares about you! This might be your partner, your mother, your sister, or your best friend. Choose people who will really listen to you, not try to tell you what to do. Just talking can help you feel a lot better.

Who would you talk to if you were upset?

1. _____

2. _____

3. _____

How do you feel now?

_____

_____

_____

What worries do you have?

_____

_____

_____

What makes you feel happy now?

_____

_____

_____

If it gets to be too much

For many pregnant women these strong emotions and worries can lead to depression* and anxiety* during pregnancy and after. If you or a family member has had mental health problems, one of these illnesses is more likely to happen in pregnancy. It can affect your health and your baby's, but you don't have to suffer.

*Depression:
A mood illness (disorder) that causes sadness or loss of interest.

Check out your feelings with the list on page 251 in Chapter 16. If you have any of these feelings, call your provider or a crisis hotline to learn more and to get help. If you have had mood problems in the past, it is really important to tell your provider.

*Anxiety (ang-zy-e-tee):
A mood disorder that causes strong worry, fear, or panic.

How much weight should I gain?

It's important to eat enough during pregnancy. But, you shouldn't eat twice as much as before you got pregnant. Most pregnant women need to eat only a little more than normal. Be sure to eat healthy foods and take prenatal vitamins. You and your baby need the best nutrition possible. See Chapter 4 for more about healthy foods.

Healthy weight gain is different for each woman

How much to gain depends on your weight before you got pregnant. Talk with your doctor or midwife about what's healthy for you. Limit your food only if he tells you to. Gaining too much weight is not healthy. Gaining too little can cause problems. The baby may be born early or be small for her age.

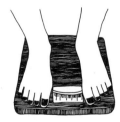

In the nine months of pregnancy, a healthy gain for a woman of normal weight would be between 25 and 35 pounds (11.5 to 16 kg). If you're very thin, your provider will want you to gain more. If you're a bit heavy, you should gain less.

Weight Gain During Pregnancy

You will gain more than just the weight of the baby. Many parts of your body will get heavier as baby grows. Look at how much each part will weigh by the end of pregnancy.

Parts of your body	Weight at delivery (average)
Baby	6–8 pounds (2.7–3.7 kg)
Uterus and amniotic fluid—where your baby grows	4 pounds (1.8 kg)
Placenta—connects mother and baby	1½ pounds (0.7 kg)
Breasts—prepare to make milk	2 pounds (0.9 kg)
Extra blood and fluid	8 pounds (3.7 kg)
Fat—stored energy for labor and breastfeeding	6 to 8 pounds (2.7–3.7 kg)

If you're pregnant with twins, you will probably gain 37 pounds (16.8 kg) or more. If you're very overweight, your provider may want you to gain as little as 15 pounds (6.8 kg) for one baby or 25 pounds (11.5 kg) for twins. This can be hard to do but will be worth it.

A note for teens

If you're a teenager, remember that your own body is still growing, too. It's very important to eat enough for you and the baby. Eat well and skip the junk food. Your provider can help you figure out what's right for you.

This is not the time to diet

If you limit the healthy foods you eat, your baby's food is limited, too. Diet pills are drugs that could be very harmful to your unborn baby. Just focus on healthy foods and exercise.

Are you afraid to gain weight? Do you diet a lot or make yourself vomit to stay thin? These habits can be very harmful to you and your baby. These are things your provider wants you to tell them. They can help.

Keeping up your healthy habits

How are you doing? You probably have been making some big changes in your life and activities. Many pregnant women must work hard to change how they eat, sleep, or exercise.

An exercise to do now: The bridge

It's never too soon to start making your tummy muscles and back stronger. Look back at Chapter 3 to review the exercises there.

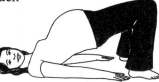

Bridge can make your tummy, back, and shoulders feel really good. Lie on your back with your knees bent. Breathe out and push with your legs to raise your bottom and back off the floor slowly. Breathe in. Then breathe out and tighten your tummy while you roll your back and bottom back to the floor slowly. Breathe in while you lie flat. Then do it again five or ten times.

It's hard to change habits

You know that smoking, drinking alcohol, or taking drugs can harm your baby. Quitting is not always easy. If you need help breaking bad habits, ask for it. Talk with your provider about getting help. There are programs to help people quit smoking, drinking, or using.

Starting new healthy habits isn't easy either. Your partner, friends, and family will want to help. But, you may have to tell them what you need.

What's been the hardest to change?

_____

_____

_____

_____

What's been the easiest to change?

_____

_____

_____

_____

Who's helping you make changes?

_____

_____

_____

_____

What healthy habits are you still working on?

_____

_____

_____

_____

Facts about partner abuse

For some people, home isn't a safe place. Partners may hit, beat, control, or yell at them. Even if they only shout or call names, it can hurt. This abuse often starts or gets worse during pregnancy.

Domestic violence is a crime. It also is a serious health problem that hurts mom, baby, and other kids in the home.

If this is happening to you, you may feel ashamed. But you're not to blame. The person who hurts you is the one who is wrong. **If you're being abused, you don't need to take it!**

There is help for you

National Domestic Violence Hotline, 800-799-7233

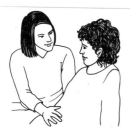

- Call the free national hotline (left). It can give you information and local contacts for shelters, counseling, and legal help.

- Tell a trusted friend, doctor or nurse, clergy member, or counselor.

- Learn about safe places to go if you need to leave your home. A women's shelter can hide you and give you protection.

If you think a friend is being abused

Do you know another woman who fears her partner? Women often hide signs of abuse. A few signs to look for are:

- ◆ Bruises or other injuries she blames on "accidents"
- ◆ Staying home alone most of the time
- ◆ Increased alcohol or drug use

Share the free hotline number on page 88. Encourage your friend to get help. It can be very hard for someone to take steps to protect herself on her own.

Common worries

Could I be having twins or multiples*?

Twins are not very likely. More than two are very rare. If your mom is a fraternal twin (not identical), you are more likely to have twins. Identical twins happen only by chance.

Tests can be done to check the number of embryos early in pregnancy. Usually they can be seen in ultrasounds.

If you are having twins or more, there are some extra risks. Your provider will talk with you about the special care you may need. With good care and healthy habits, you are very likely to have healthy babies.

Things that may happen with twins or multiples:

- ◆ Gain more weight than with a single baby
- ◆ Need more rest (lying on your left side is best)
- ◆ Have more checkups later in pregnancy
- ◆ Go into preterm labor (see Chapter 8)
- ◆ Need a c-section

*Multiples: Two or more babies.

Twins love to be close to each other, like they were in the womb.

Could I lose my baby?

Some pregnancies end on their own in the first five months. This is called a miscarriage or spontaneous abortion. Many take place in the first trimester. It can happen before you are sure you're pregnant. But it can be a very sad time. They are not caused by doing normal things. You can work hard, go jogging, and have sex

---

Warning Signs of Miscarriage

Know how to reach your doctor, midwife, or nurse at all hours.
Call if any of these things happen:

◆ Bleeding from your vagina

◆ Painful cramps in your belly or back

◆ A jelly-like blob coming from your vagina. (If this happens, save it in a plastic bag for him to see.)

---

with no need to worry. An early miscarriage often happens if something is wrong with the baby. It might not have attached to your uterus and started to grow. Or, the growing baby might have something very wrong with it.

Some miscarriages happen because of mom's health problems. This might be an infection, a problem in the uterus, or a very bad injury. Some drugs, chemicals, and foods make miscarriage more likely.

You usually can't stop a miscarriage once it starts. And you may never know what made it happen. The best thing to do is take really good care of yourself. Go back to Chapters 2, 3, and 4 to review the ways you can try to avoid a miscarriage.

How do I know I'm having a miscarriage?

Miscarriage can happen in the first few weeks of pregnancy. It may seem like a late, heavy menstrual period.

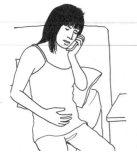

If miscarriage happens after the first month, you will have heavy bleeding and cramps. A bloody blob may come out of your vagina. (Keep it for your provider.) Be sure to call your provider. He will want to check to see what is happening. He may do a pelvic exam, ultrasound, and other tests.

After a miscarriage

Your provider should check your uterus. It's important to make sure that there's nothing left in your womb. That could cause infection. Talk with your provider about what might have led to the miscarriage. It is not always easy to find the answer.

You may feel very sad for weeks or months after this happens. These feelings are very natural. Other people may not understand your sadness. It often helps to talk to other women who have miscarried. Tell your provider how you feel.

After you heal, you will probably be able to get pregnant again. Many women have a normal pregnancy after a miscarriage. Ask how soon to try again. Do you need to prepare at all? Meanwhile, keep your body healthy.

Why do I need an HIV test?

Pregnant women are usually checked for HIV. This is because many people who have HIV don't know it. It's very important, even if you think it's not possible. Your provider should talk with you about the test before and after you take it. Be sure to ask about the test if you are worried.

If a woman has HIV, her doctor will help make sure she and her baby get the right care. There are drugs to help mom stay well. There are also ways to protect the baby from getting HIV in the womb or at birth.

Could my baby have a birth defect?

A small number of babies are born with birth defects*. Some are serious, but others are not. Some can be found before birth, but others cannot.

*Birth defect:
A health condition that is there from birth.

Does anyone in your family have a birth defect? If so, talk with a genetics counselor as soon as possible. There are tests that you can have during pregnancy to look for some birth defects.

What can cause a birth defect?

- A health problem in mom. (Example: If a mother has rubella (German measles) in early pregnancy, her baby might have hearing, heart, and eye problems.)

- Something that gets into the mom's body and harms the baby. (Example: Alcohol can cause serious defects as the brain and body develop.)

- A problem that happens during birth. (Example: Too little oxygen for the baby during delivery could cause brain damage.)

Tests in first trimester

Test	What is it for?	How is it done?	Risks or side effects
Ultrasound *At first, second, or third visit*	Confirm pregnancy, learn age of baby, and check for twins	Ultrasound in your vagina or on your belly	None
Cystic Fibrosis (CF) screen *Anytime*	Find out if both parents have the CF gene	DNA test — blood or mouth swab (mom and dad)	None
First trimester screen ("triple screen") *11 to 13 weeks*	Check for possible Down syndrome and Trisomy 18	Blood test (mom) and ultrasound	None
Cell-free fetal DNA testing ("noninvasive prenatal testing") *After 10 weeks*	Check for some genetic disorders, like Down syndrome, Trisomy 13, or Trisomy 18	Blood test (mom)	None
Chorionic villus sampling (CVS) *10 to 12 weeks*	Diagnose some genetic disorders, like Down syndrome or CF	A small piece of the placenta is taken	Small chance of miscarriage, blood problems, or infection

- ♦ A "genetic" defect that comes from a parent's genes. (Example: Sicklecell disease is a genetic disease that can be passed down from parent to child.)

- ♦ Unknown causes. Many defects are mysteries.

Prenatal screening and testing for defects

Some basic tests are given to all women at the beginning of pregnancy. These check for infections, blood problems, and immunities. Most providers offer other screening tests in the third and fourth month. These check for possible birth defects and other health problems. Some are required, others are not.

If any of these tests shows a possible problem, more tests will be done. Often these tests will find there is no problem. If there really is a problem, your provider would talk with you and your partner. He might send you to a specialist.

Genetic testing

If you know someone in your family has genetic problems, ask your provider which tests would be most helpful. Learn about the tests so you can decide if you want them. If your baby has a defect, it's helpful to know early. This gives you and your providers time to prepare.

You may ask to see a genetic counselor. Check your health insurance plan to find out what genetic services are covered.

After birth, all babies in the U.S. are also screened (tested) for genetic problems that are rare but serious. Finding these problems early means the baby can get the best care right away. See Chapter 11 for more on newborn screening.

Tips for partners

- Be prepared for your partner to be more emotional than usual. Try to go with her ups and downs.
- Be prepared for your partner to feel much more tired than before.
- Help out when she feels exhausted. Take over some chores she normally does herself.
- If a miscarriage happens, be as understanding as you can. It could feel like a very big deal to your partner. Just tell her you're sorry. It may not help to tell her she can have another baby.

Month-to-month checkups

Your first prenatal visit

Your doctor or midwife will give you a complete checkup (exam). At this visit, he will usually:

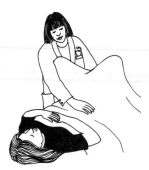

- Ask you about your health history and habits. Tell him as much as you can, even things you may not like to talk about. Things that don't seem important to you might make a difference in your care. The more your provider knows, the better care he can give you.

- Ask about the health of your parents and relatives. Some health conditions of family members could affect your health and your pregnancy.

- Measure your height, weight, temperature, heart rate, and blood pressure.

- Check your breasts and listen to your lungs.

- Do a pelvic exam to find out the size and position of your uterus. A pelvic exam is done by putting the fingers of one hand into the vagina and pressing on your belly with the other. He may also look at the cervix and do a Pap test*.

*Pap test:
A lab test to show signs of cervical cancer. Also called a "Pap smear."

- Look at your tiny baby using an ultrasound in your vagina (transvaginal ultrasound). This helps figure out how far along you are. (Later ultrasounds will be done on your belly.)

- Get blood, urine, and other samples to learn more about your health. Your provider needs to know about diseases like chlamydia, hepatitis B, and HIV as soon as possible.

- Give you a prescription for prenatal vitamins.

All about me (things to tell your provider)

I am _____ years old. My birthday is _____.
(month, day, year)

I am _____ inches tall and weighed _____ pounds/kg before I got pregnant.

My last period started on _____.
(date)

- Health problems I have (illnesses, surgeries, etc.):

  _____

  _____

  _____

- Health problems in my family, my partner, my other children, my parents, brothers, sisters:

  _____

  _____

  _____

- Medicines, herbs, and supplements I use:

  _____

  _____

  _____

- Questions I have about being pregnant:

  _____

  _____

  _____

First prenatal checkup notes

(Write down what happens at each checkup to help you remember.)

Date _____ (usually 4 to 8 weeks after your last period).

I am about _____ weeks pregnant today.

I weigh _____ pounds/kg.

My blood pressure is _____.

Tests I had today:

_____

_____

_____

_____

My provider's name is

_____

Phone number:_____

Emergency phone number:_____

Email address: _____

Things I learned today:

1. My baby's "due date" _____

_____

2. _____

_____

_____

3. _____

_____

_____

My next checkup will be on

The _____ of _____, at ___:___.
    (date)   **(month)**   **(time)**

Month 3

After the first visit, most checkups will be simpler and shorter. Your weight, blood pressure, and the size of your uterus will be measured. You may be asked to give a urine sample. Your provider will check your baby's heartbeat. (Soon you'll be able to hear it, too.) Be sure to ask any questions you have.

At some visits, you will have ultrasound pictures taken to see how the baby is growing. You'll be able to see your baby on the screen. It often is possible to see a tiny penis and know the sex of the baby.

Some new parents don't want to know baby's sex before birth. Be sure to tell your provider and the ultrasound technician if you don't want to know. Otherwise, they might tell you.

Questions you may want to ask at your three-month checkup

- *What can I do if I am constipated?*
- *Why do I feel so happy one day and so sad the next?*
- *Am I gaining enough weight?*
- *How will I know if I am having twins?*
- *I am having trouble quitting smoking. What will make stopping easier?*

Other questions I have:

1._____

2._____

3._____

4._____

5._____

6._____

Three-month checkup notes

On this date, _____, I had my three-month visit.

I am _____ weeks pregnant.

I weigh _____ pounds/kg now.

I have gained _____ pounds/kg since my last checkup.

My blood pressure is _____.

Things I learned today:

1. _____

_____

_____

2. _____

_____

_____

3. _____

_____

_____

My next checkup will be on

The _____ of _____, at ___:___.
    (date)   **(month)**   **(time)**

Chapter 8

Second Trimester: Months 4, 5, and 6

Weeks 13 to 28

Your body is getting used to having a baby growing inside. You probably will feel better in this trimester than before. You may have more energy and less morning sickness.

Your body will really change shape now. Exercise becomes more and more important. Strengthen your back and belly to hold your growing baby.

It can be very exciting to feel the baby move. At 20 weeks, you are half-way through your pregnancy. Now is the time to sign up for a childbirth class. Take one that will end before your ninth month starts.

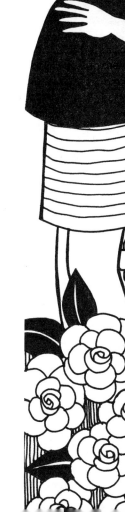

Look in this chapter for:

Weeks 13 to 28, page 99
How your baby is growing
How your body is changing
Tuning up your body for life, page 102
Keeping that loving feeling, page 104
Help for common problems, page 105
Important medical things to know, page 108
Warning signs—Preterm labor, page 110
Tips for partners, page 111
Month-to-month checkups, page 112

How your baby is growing

Your baby in month 4 (13 to 17 weeks)

Babies can feel touch and hear sounds by 4 months. So press on your belly when your baby moves and talk to him. He will know you care about him.

- At the end of this month, your baby will be up to 7 inches long.
- He will weigh 4 to 5 ounces, like a small can of tuna.
- His bones and muscles are forming.
- He has skin that is almost see-through.
- He is able to suck and swallow.
- His very first poop is already forming.

Month 5 (18 to 23 weeks)

- At the end of this month, your baby will be about 10 inches long. That is around half as long as most newborns.
- He will weigh 1/2 to 1 pound, less than a small can of beans.
- His skin is very wrinkly. It's covered in a thick white cream called vernix.
- He kicks, rolls, and flips often. You can finally feel him moving! If not, tell your provider.
- He can hear.
- His fingernails are getting long.
- He has hair on his head and fine hair called lanugo on his body. He has eyebrows and eyelashes.

Month 6 (24 to 28 weeks)

- At the end of this month, your baby will be up to 12 inches long. That is about the length of your arm from elbow to hand.
- Your baby will weigh about 1½ to 2 pounds. This is as much as a half-gallon of milk.
- He lies curled up, his knees against his chest. His head may be up, down or sideward.
- His eyes are almost done forming. He can open and close his eyes.

- He has taste buds, fingerprints, and footprints.
- He has asleep and awake times. He can be startled.
- Genitals are formed. A boy's testicles are coming down toward the penis. A girl's organs are formed and all of the eggs she'll have in her life are in her ovaries.

How your body is changing

Your body in month 4 (13 to 17 weeks)

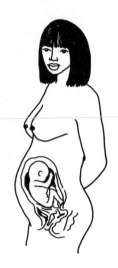

- You are starting to gain weight more quickly. You should gain about 1 pound each week from now on.
- Morning sickness will likely end. You will start to feel hungry more often.
- Your breasts may be less sore than before.
- You may not need to go to the bathroom as often.
- You might feel your baby move, like a little flutter or a gas bubble. If not, don't worry. It's still early.
- Your belly starts to show and you may need to wear bigger clothes and bras.

Month 5 (18 to 23 weeks)

- By week 20 you should feel your baby move often. If not, tell your provider.
- The top of your uterus may be up to your belly button.
- Your face may get light or dark patches. A dark line may run down the middle of your belly. These changes should go away after your baby is born.
- You may have pains in your sides, hips, and thighs from your growing belly.
- You may have some swelling and tingling in your hands and feet.

Month 6 (24 to 28 weeks)

- The top of your uterus is now above your belly button.
- The skin on your belly, breasts, hands, and feet may itch.

- You may start to feel your uterus contracting and relaxing.
- You may get stretch marks on your belly and breasts.
- Your belly button may pop out.
- Your legs may get cramps and your ankles may swell.
- The areolas around your nipples may look bigger and darker.

Tuning up your body for life

Our bodies are made for moving, not sitting still. When you are active, you help your muscles. Remember this when you are reaching up to a high shelf or sweeping the floor.

If you have to sit most of the day at work, get up every hour for just a few minutes. Move around, even if you stay at your desk. Walk while you talk on the phone. If you are watching TV, get up during commercials. Moving around is one of the best healthy habits to do throughout your life.

Walking for overall health

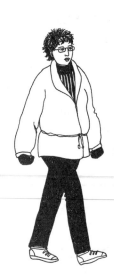

- Take a half-hour walk every day. You don't have to do it all at once. Wear comfortable sport shoes. For the best workout, go fast, but not so fast that you can't talk. Swing your arms to exercise your upper body.
- Take walks in different places so you don't get bored. Invite a friend to the mall or a park. When you walk alone, listen to music or a book.
- Walk tall. Hold your belly in and your shoulders back.

Exercises to help you get ready for birth

Birth will be easier if you are in good shape. Remember the exercises in Chapter 3. They will help your core to be strong for birth. Here are some more to do every day.

Kegel squeeze helps hold up your uterus

This exercise strengthens the muscles around your vagina. These muscles help hold up the weight of your baby and uterus. They also help you control your urine (pee). After birth, the Kegel squeeze helps keep your vagina and bladder strong. This exercise will help you even as you get older.

An easy way to learn to do the Kegel squeeze is while you are peeing on the toilet. Here's how:

1. Squeeze the muscles you use to stop your pee. These are muscles around your vagina and perineum*. This is called the Kegel squeeze. Try **not** to use your stomach muscles or buttocks.

2. Hold tight while you count 1–2–3–4–5.

3. Relax, and then squeeze again. (Once you know how this exercise feels, don't do it on the toilet.)

*Perineum: The skin and tissue between the vagina and anus.

You can do Kegels anywhere. Try it standing at the kitchen sink or waiting for the bus. Practice until you can do it 25 times, three or four times a day.

Squats help strengthen your core

Squatting strengthens your tummy, legs, and back. It also stretches your hips and the joints of your pelvis. Being able to squat helps a lot when you carry the extra weight of your baby inside. The stretching will help baby come through the birth canal.

Here's how to practice squatting:

1. Stand facing a chair with feet apart.

2. Pull your tummy in and keep your back as straight as possible.

3. Bend your knees and squat down slowly, holding onto the chair. (Don't do this if your knees hurt.)

4. Rise up slowly, keeping your shoulders back.

5. Do this slowly 5 or 10 times.

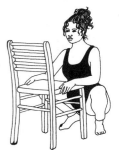

Squat holding onto a chair for balance.

Learning to lift safely

Learning to squat will protect your back later. It is the safest way to lift heavy things. You will be doing a lot of lifting as your baby grows.

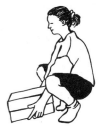

Lifting safely by squatting with back straight.

Sitting with knees spread

Stretching helps you spread your hips and knees wide apart during birth. Here's an easy way to stretch while you are relaxing:

1. Sit on the floor with your back straight.
2. Put the soles of your feet together.
3. Spread your knees wide apart and keep them there for a minute or two.
4. Pull your knees together, then spread them wide again.

Healthy snacks to remember

- **Fresh fruits**—orange, apple, peach, or papaya with non-fat, non-sweetened yogurt on top. Add chopped walnuts for crunch.
- **Trail mix**—raisins, apricots, or prunes mixed with pumpkin seeds, peanuts, or almonds.
- **Raw vegetables**—carrots, tomatoes, or broccoli to dip in hummus or yogurt.
- **Whole grains**—bread or crackers with peanut butter.
- **Water**—instead of sodas or too much coffee.

Keeping that loving feeling

Having sex is safe and healthy in a normal pregnancy. Your provider will tell you not to have sex if there is reason to worry.

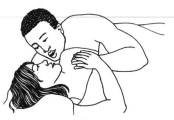

The changes happening to you can mean sex and intimacy feel different. Some women want to have a lot of sex at this time. Other women don't want to have any at all.

Tell your partner how you're feeling. Ask what he or she is feeling, too. There are many ways to enjoy sex. Talk about what you think might feel good. Try different positions, like lying on your side with your partner behind you. Try other ways of being close, like cuddling or massaging each other.

If you don't want to have sex, say so. Remind each other that pregnancy doesn't last forever.

When you do have sex, it is safest for you and baby if you only have sex with someone who is only having sex with you. Be sure to use a condom if either of you has had sex with someone else. That will help prevent you from getting an STD that could hurt your baby. If any fluid or blood comes from your vagina, stop having sex and call your provider right away.

Spending time with older children

If you have other kids, make sure you spend time with them. Talk about the baby who is coming. Read some books together about new babies. Give both boys and girls a doll so they will have their own baby. All these things will help make this big change seem more real. Let them know that you will still love them after the baby is born. Some practical tips:

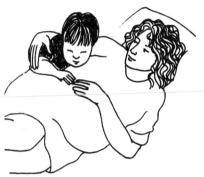

- If you plan to move a child into a different room, do it a few months before the baby is born.

- Get some larger clothes for them now. That way, you will not have to go out shopping too soon after baby comes.

Help for common problems

How to cool heartburn?

Heartburn* after eating is common in pregnancy. These tips might help you feel better:

- Eat smaller meals, more often.

- Chew your food well.

- Stop eating foods that make it worse. Spicy or greasy foods are common causes.

- Wait 1 to 3 hours after eating to go to bed.

- Lie down with your head and back propped up a bit.

- Wear clothes that are loose around your waist.

If these things don't work, ask your provider what medicines you can take safely to help you feel better.

*Heartburn: Sharp or burning chest pains from acid backing up into the tube that goes from your mouth to your stomach.

What to do about swollen feet and ankles?

Are your ankles and feet swollen? Some swelling is normal in pregnancy. You should keep drinking plenty of water. Here are some other ways to help:

- Wear support hose and shoes with low heels.
- Lie on the bed with your legs higher that your head. Put your feet up against the wall or up on pillows.
- Move your legs often, pointing your toes, and making circles with your feet.
- Put one foot up on a low stool or box when you have to stand.
- Sleep on your left side.
- Stay away from salty foods, caffeine, and diet sodas
- Swim or do exercises in a swimming pool.

Sudden swelling is a warning sign. Call your provider right away.

How can you deal with varicose veins?

Many women get swollen blue (varicose) veins during pregnancy. These veins are most common in your legs, but can also happen around your vagina. Varicose veins are often painless, but can get quite sore. Here are ways to prevent them or keep them from getting worse. They usually go away a little while after baby is born.

- Walk every day. Exercising your leg muscles helps to keep the blood flowing well in your veins.
- Put your feet up when you sit down.
- Take breaks and change position often when you sit or stand for a long time.
- Wear support hose and comfortable shoes.

If you have varicose veins around your vagina, ask your provider about getting a special sling (support garment).

How to care for hemorrhoids in your bottom?

Hemorroids are swollen veins in your anus and rectum that can itch, hurt, or bleed. They often can get worse if you often have to strain (push hard) to have bowel movements.

To feel better, wipe the area with witch hazel* pads. Soaking in a warm bath can also feel good. Talk to your provider if you think you have hemorrhoids.

The best way to keep from having hemorrhoids is to keep your stools (poop) soft. (See below for tips on preventing constipation.)

*Witch hazel:
A soothing, safe natural remedy available at drug stores. It comes in a bottle or on pads.

Are your nipples shaped right for breastfeeding?

If your nipples don't stick out naturally you don't need to worry. You can still breastfeed.

Some women's nipples are flat. Try squeezing them around the edge of the areola (dark area). If they do not stick out more when you squeeze, they are inverted.

Some women's nipples stick out more as pregnancy goes on. If they do not, there are simple things to do when you start breastfeeding. You can use a device to pull out the nipple. Your nurse or breastfeeding consultant can help you get started.

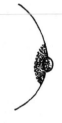
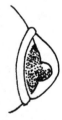

Nipple shell

How can you relieve breast pain?

As your breasts get bigger and heavier, they may hurt. A bra that fits well will keep them as comfortable as possible. You may want a stronger bra for during the day and a stretchy bra to wear at home or at night.

How can you cope with constipation*?

Constipation is very uncomfortable during pregnancy. Here are some tips to keep stools soft:

*Constipation:
Bowel movements that don't come at least every 2 or 3 days. They are very dry and hard.

- ◆ Exercise every day.
- ◆ Drink 8 to 10 tall glasses of liquids every day; at least half should be water.
- ◆ Eat foods with lots of fiber, such as fresh fruits and vegetables, whole grain cereal and bread, and beans.
- ◆ Snack on dried prunes or apricots each day.

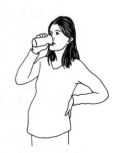

- Get plenty of rest and time with loved ones. Stress and worry can make constipation worse.

If you get constipated often, try drinking warm prune juice. Ask your provider if you should take extra fiber or a stool softener.

Important medical things to know

Diabetes in pregnancy

Some women get diabetes (gestational diabetes—sometimes called GDM or DM) while they are pregnant. DM can cause serious problems for both mom and baby.

Your provider will test your blood for this condition around 26 to 28 weeks. If that test is too high, she may want to do another test to be sure. If that comes back high, she'll help you learn how to control it. Most women can do this with careful eating and exercise. Some need medicines. This kind of diabetes usually goes away after birth.

Anyone can get GDM, but it is most likely if you are:

- Over age 25
- Very overweight
- Have family members with diabetes
- Are African American, Hispanic, Native American, Alaska Native, Asian, Native Hawaiian, or Pacific Islander
- Have had a baby over 9 pounds or an unexplained stillborn baby

Your Rh factor

Early in your pregnancy, your provider will check your blood type. Part of this test is the Rh (Rhesus) factor. Most women are Rh positive. The baby's father's blood may need to be tested, too. This helps predict baby's blood type.

If your blood is Rh negative and baby's is positive, there could be problems later on. Your blood may make cells to attack baby's blood. This doesn't usually happen until birth, so this baby is

Tests in the second trimester

Test	What is it for?	How is it done?	Risks or side effects
Maternal Blood Screen 15 to 20 weeks	Check for birth defects, like Down syndrome and heart defects	Blood test (mom)	None
Amniocentesis ("amnio") 15 to 20 weeks	Check for genetic conditions, like Down syndrome	Amniotic fluid is taken by a long needle.	Chance of cramping, bleeding, or leaking. Small chance of miscarriage
Ultrasound 18 to 20 weeks	See how baby is growing and check for birth defects.	Ultrasound on belly (See pages 77 and 97)	None
Glucose screen 24 to 28 weeks	Check for gestational diabetes (See page 108)	Blood test (mom)	Mild upset stomach, dizziness, headache

likely safe. But, if you get pregnant with another Rh positive baby, that baby could be in great danger.

Your provider will give you a shot of RhIg (Rh immunoglobulin) at 28 weeks. This keeps baby safe during birth. If your baby is Rh positive, you will get another shot of RhIg after you give birth. This will protect any future babies you may have.

Braxton-Hicks contractions

Soon you will start to feel your uterus contracting. Your whole belly will get hard for a moment and then relax. These are called Braxton-Hicks contractions. They are normal and help your body get ready for real labor. They can feel strange, but they don't usually hurt. They start and stop a lot and don't get stronger. They will happen more as you get closer to your due date.

Preterm labor

When real labor starts before 37 weeks, it's called preterm labor. It is very serious. Often it can be stopped to give the baby more time to grow inside.

Every day a baby stays inside your uterus helps him be better prepared for life outside. A baby born too early is more likely to

Warning Signs—Preterm Labor

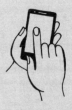

Call your doctor or midwife right away if you have any of these signs:

- Bleeding or pink or brown fluid coming from your vagina
- Loss of the mucus plug or clear fluid leaking from the vagina
- Contractions every 10 minutes or less, or cramps like those during your period
- Low back ache that may be steady or come and go
- Heavy feeling in your pelvis and vagina, like the baby is pushing down
- Unusual tightness or hardness of your belly
- A general feeling that something is wrong

have health problems. At 24 weeks (6 months), a baby may survive, but would need lots of special care.

It is important to know the signs of preterm labor on the next page. These signs do not always mean preterm labor has started. However, it is best to call your health care provider right away.

Your doctor or midwife may want you to come in as soon as you can. Or she may ask you to lie on your left side and rest for an hour first. She may ask you to drink a few glasses of water or juice. Sometimes these things are enough to stop the contractions.

Some women are more likely to have preterm labor than others. Be sure to call your provider right away if you:

- Have had a preterm baby before
- Are expecting more than one baby
- Are very stressed or afraid
- Have gum disease
- Have an infection or vaginal disease (UTI, chlamydia, bacterial vaginosis)
- Have been smoking or using alcohol or drugs

Tips for partners

You are essential to your unborn baby's life, birth, and growth. Here are some things to do as you wait for birth.

Practical things

- Go to prenatal visits when you can.
- If you will be a birth partner, go to birth classes. Practice the relaxation exercises together between classes.
- If you think you do not want to watch the birth, say so. You could help during labor and then leave the room when the birth stage starts.
- Pick out a car seat together. (See Chapters 6 and 14.) Read the directions and practice buckling it in the car.
- Talk together about names for your baby.

Show these tips to your partner, if he hasn't read the whole book!

Feelings

- Take time together. Do things now that will be harder after baby is born. Take a vacation. Get plenty of sleep.
- Hold your hand on your partner's tummy. Feel your baby move. Tell him what you will do when he's here.
- Pay attention to your and your partner's moods. Watch out for depression and anxiety.

Sex now

- If the pregnancy is going well, having sex won't harm baby. However, your pregnant partner may not enjoy it as much as the baby gets bigger.
- Use positions that are comfortable for her.
- Do not have sex if your partner is bleeding, the bag of waters has broken, or she is having preterm labor. If those things happen, anything put in her vagina could cause infection.

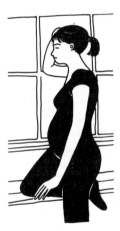

Watch out for mood changes. Hormones and lack of sleep can make these feelings much worse.

If you feel left out by your partner at this time, talk about it. She may be focused on your baby. Talking with each other about feelings is a good habit.

Month-to-month checkups
Month 4
Questions to ask at your four-month visit

- *Is my blood pressure normal?*
- *Can I keep exercising?*
- *I have not felt my baby move yet. Is she okay?*
- *If I have had a c-section before, must I have one again?*

Other questions you have:

1. _____

_____

2. _____

_____

Your four-month checkup notes

On this date, _____, I had my four-month visit.

I am ___ weeks pregnant.

I weigh ___ pounds/kg now.

I have gained ___ pounds/kg since my last checkup.

I have gained ___ pounds/kg since I got pregnant.

My blood pressure is _____.

Things I learned today:

1. _____

_____

2. _____

_____

Your next visit will be on

The _____ of _____, at _____:_____.
      (date)   **(month)**   **(time)**

Month 5
Questions to ask at your five-month visit

- *Is my baby growing well?*
- *Is there any chance I could be having twins?*
- *Where can I find a good childbirth class?*
- *How long should I keep on working?*
- *Is my blood pressure normal?*
- *What can I do about varicose veins?*

Other questions you have:

1. _____

   _____

2. _____

   _____

Your five-month checkup notes

On this date, _____, I had my five-month visit.

I am ___ weeks pregnant.   I weigh ___ pounds/kg now.

I have gained ___ pounds/kg since my last checkup.

I have gained ___ pounds/kg since I got pregnant.

My blood pressure is _____.

Things I learned today:

1. _____

   _____

2. _____

   _____

Your next visit will be on

The _____ of _____, at _____:_____.
    (date)   **(month)**   **(time)**

Month 6
Questions to ask at your six-month visit:

- *What can I do to get ready for breastfeeding?*
- *Am I likely to go into preterm labor?*
- *Why does my baby move a lot some days and not much on others?*
- *How do I know if I am getting enough exercise?*
- *Is my blood Rh negative?*
- *When will I have the test for gestational diabetes?*

Other questions you have:

1. _____

  _____

2. _____

  _____

Your six-month checkup notes

On this date, _____, I had my six-month visit.

I am ___ weeks pregnant.

I weigh ___ pounds/kg now.

I have gained ___ pounds/kg since my last checkup.

I have gained ___ pounds/kg since I got pregnant.

My blood pressure is _____.

Things I learned today:

1. _____

  _____

2. _____

  _____

Chapter 9

Third Trimester: Months 7, 8, and 9

29 to 40 weeks

Your third trimester is starting. You have done a lot to help your baby be healthy. Your pregnancy is almost over. Are you eager to meet baby?

For months, your body has been getting ready for birth. Now is the time to read Chapter 10. Go to a childbirth class.

Most important: Look back at page 110 in Chapter 8 to be sure you know the signs of preterm labor. You may be getting tired of being pregnant, but your baby should stay safely inside your body until at least 39 weeks, if possible.

Look in this chapter for:

29 to 40 weeks, page 115
 How your baby is growing
 How your body is changing
Third trimester basics, page 118
 Exercises, What if you can't sleep
 Tests you need now
Warning signs—High blood pressure, page 120
Your body getting ready for labor, page 122
Make your birth plan, page 126
Tips for partners, page 127
**Month-to-month checkups,
 page 128**

How your baby is growing

Your baby in month 7 (29 to 32 weeks)

- ◆ At the end of this month, your baby will be up to 16 inches (40 cm) long. She will weigh about 3 pounds (1.3 kg).

- ◆ Her body is well formed. She would have a good chance of living if she were born now. But, she would need lots of care.

- ◆ You may feel her hiccup. She can even suck her thumb!

- ◆ She can blink and react to light and noise.

Month 8 (33 to 36 weeks)

- ◆ Your baby will be about 18 inches (45 cm) long and weigh about 5 pounds (2.3 kg).

- ◆ Her brain still has a lot of growing to do. It is only 2/3 as big as it will be at 40 weeks.

- ◆ She may move a bit less. There is less room to roll around inside the uterus now. Tell your provider if baby moves a lot less.

- ◆ Her kicks and stretches may push your belly out so you can see her move. Can you feel her back, foot, or elbow?

Month 9 (37 to 40 weeks)

- ◆ Most babies are about 19 to 21 inches (48 to 53 cm) long at birth. Most weigh 6 to 9 pounds (2.7 to 4 kg).

- ◆ Her lungs are still getting ready to breathe air.

- ◆ She is still safest in your body until at least 39 weeks.

- ◆ She is gaining fat to help her stay warm.

- ◆ She is crowded in the uterus, but you should still feel her kick and roll.

- ◆ Her fingernails are getting longer.

- ◆ She will settle down lower in your uterus. It could be with her head down, or her bottom down (breech), or laying on her side.

How your body is changing

Your body in month 7 (29 to 32 weeks)

- You could gain another 4 pounds (1.8 kg) this month.
- You should still feel baby roll around. If she's moving a lot less, call your provider.
- Your feet and legs may swell. If your hands and face swell a lot, call your provider.
- It may be hard to keep your balance with your big belly. Be careful not to fall.
- You may feel very warm and have a hard time sleeping.
- You will probably feel Braxton-Hicks contractions.

Month 8 (33 to 36 weeks)

- You will gain about 4 more pounds (1.8 kg) this month.
- Baby will push into your ribs.
- She will also push your stomach, lungs, and other organs aside. It may be hard to take a deep breath or eat a big meal.
- Your breasts may swell more and get sore. Colostrum may leak from your nipples.
- You may feel very warm. Wear light, loose clothes.
- You may leak urine when you sneeze, cough, or laugh.
- Your hip joints are getting looser and may ache. You may feel dizzy if you stand up suddenly. Try not to fall.

Month 9 (37 to 40 weeks)

- You will gain about 4 more pounds (1.8 kg) this month.
- The baby will move down (drop) into your pelvis. She is getting into position for birth. You may feel like your uterus is pushing down on your cervix or bottom.
- Breathing and eating may be easier after this, but you may need to urinate more often. You also may get constipated more easily.
- Your cervix starts to get soft and thin before it opens.
- You may feel heavy and tired. Take time to rest.

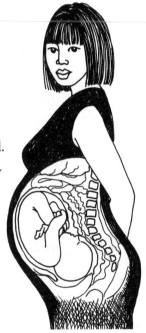

In the last three months, the growing baby pushes against your lungs, stomach, and intestines.

Third trimester basics

Your to-do list

- Go to your prenatal checkups. You will have two in your eighth month and more in your last month.

"Just before my baby was born, I cleaned all the kitchen cabinets completely. I was amazed that I had the energy for it."

- Go to your childbirth classes. Ask your birth partner to go with you. Practice the exercises that you learn.

- Make your birth plan (later in this chapter). Talk it over with your provider at a checkup.

- Choose your baby's provider. (See Chapter 5.)

- Learn about baby care. Your hospital, clinic, or community center may have classes. You won't have much time after baby is born.

Healthy habits–Keep 'em up!

- Continue to cook and eat healthy food like protein, veggies, and grains. And remember your prenatal vitamins.

- Drink at least 8 tall glasses of water each day.

- Take a walk each day, even if it is a slow one.

- Stay away from alcohol, drugs, cigarettes, and smoke. Avoid people or places that make you feel unsafe.

- When driving, try to sit as far as possible from the steering wheel. If you are very short, this is really important.

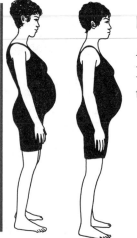

NO!   YES!

Practice standing tall and pulling in your belly.

Exercises to do now

As your belly gets bigger, make sure you don't give up on exercise. Look back at the exercises in Chapters 3, 7, and 8. Make sure to do these two:

- Now it is more important than ever to keep your back strong, stand up straight, and pull in your belly. A growing baby will make your belly heavier. It will be easy to let it hang out.

- Stretching your hips will really help get you ready for birth. So practice now by sitting this way for a while every day. Try it on the floor or sitting on a firm chair without arms.

Sit on the floor to stretch your hips.

What to do if you can't sleep

It can be really hard to get good sleep in these months. As your baby gets bigger, it is harder to get comfortable. Your back and neck may ache. Your legs may cramp and your hips may hurt. It can be hard to breathe well and you may have heartburn. You probably need to get up often to go to the bathroom.

Try to be active every day. Even just a walk after dinner can help you sleep better. Try these tips for getting more rest:

◆ Nap when you can. Your body needs all the rest it can get right now.

◆ When settling down to rest, take deep breaths. Practice relaxation in the ways you learned in childbirth class.

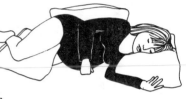

◆ Lie on your left side. Put pillows under your back, belly, and neck. Add a big pillow between your knees.

Get comfortable—lie on your left side with pillows under your knee.

◆ Avoid lying flat on your back for very long. This can be bad for you and baby.

◆ Drink most of your water early in the day. Drink less later. This can help you get up less often to pee at night.

◆ Notice how you are feeling. Not sleeping could be a sign of depression or anxiety. (See Chapter 16.)

Baby's kicks and naps

Babies have quiet and active times each day. You probably will feel your baby move at least 10 times in 1 to 2 hours. As you get closer to the birth, she may slow down. She doesn't have much room in there to move.

If you think baby has been moving a lot less for 24 hours, call your provider. He may want to check on her to find out why.

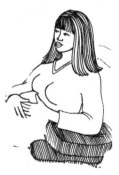

Feeling baby move

Important medical questions

What if my blood pressure is high?

High blood pressure during pregnancy (also called toxemia, preeclampsia, or gestational hypertension) can become dangerous to you and your baby. It is most likely to happen with a first pregnancy. If your blood pressure is high, you will need to take special care of yourself to prevent more serious problems.

Signs that your blood pressure may be getting worse

- Sudden weight gain (more than a pound in a day)
- Headache
- Swollen hands and face
- Blurred vision or seeing spots
- Nausea and vomiting

This could be an emergency. Call your doctor or midwife right away!

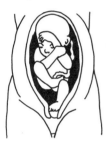

Baby in breech position with one leg down

What if my baby's head isn't down?

Almost all babies are head-down and facing mom's back before birth. (This is called the vertex position.) This is the best position for birth. It is easiest for baby to move down and out head first. But your baby might be head-down, head-up (breech), or sideways (transverse). She may also be facing your back (posterior) or front (anterior). In these other positions, birth through the vagina would be hard. In many cases, a mom may need a c-section.

What prenatal tests do I need now?

Test	What is it for?	How is it done?	Risks or side effects
Biophysical Profile ("BPP") *Can be done any time. Often done if mom goes past her due date.*	Check baby's breathing, movement, muscle tone, and heart rate. Also checks amniotic fluid level.	Ultrasound and nonstress test (see below)	None
Nonstress test *After 28 weeks*	Look for any signs of distress in baby	A belt around mom's belly measures baby's heart rate	None
Group B streptococcus *36–37 weeks*	Check for group B strep bacteria and risk of infection to baby	Swab from vagina and anus	None

Ways you can help baby turn over

If your baby doesn't have her head down by 34 to 36 weeks, you may try to help her turn. Here are some gentle things you can do that might help to get her to flip.

- Try poses that open the pelvis and give space to baby to turn herself (breech tilt, sidelying, and sifting)
- Chiropractic care (Webster Technique)
- Massage or craniosacral work (Maya Massage or myofascial Release)
- Sound, cold, relaxation (hypnosis, journaling, rest)
- Homeopathic remedy (moxibustion)

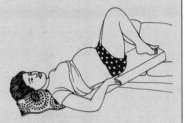

Breech tilt is a way to give baby space to turn naturally. Lie head down on a propped up ironing board.

These are not proven, but many women have found them helpful. Ask your provider if there's any reason why not to try any of these. See Chapter 17 for resources to learn more.

If baby is not head-down as your due date gets closer, you can try gentle ways to get her to turn (see box above). Or your doctor or midwife may try to get her to turn by pushing on the outside of your uterus. This is called an external version. He would press his hands on the outside of your belly to carefully push your baby into a new position. He'll watch baby's heart rate while he's pushing to make sure it doesn't upset her too much. It doesn't feel good, but it can help you avoid surgery.

If your provider doesn't turn your baby or other measures don't work, your provider would likely say that a c-section is safest. See Chapter 10 to learn about c-section.

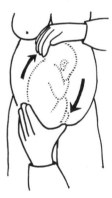

An external version to change baby's position

Do I want to have my son circumcised?

This is up to you and your partner to decide. At birth, the skin on the penis (foreskin) is intact. It covers all the way over the tip. Circumcision is a surgery that cuts part of this skin off, so the tip of the penis is not covered. If you choose to have it done, it will be done soon after birth. So, it is good to decide before baby comes. Learn more about circumcision in Chapter 11.

Your body getting ready for labor

Pre-labor contractions

The mild Braxton-Hicks contractions you may have been feeling will get stronger closer to the birth. Sometimes these contractions feel so strong that you might think they are the real thing. They may be called "false labor." If you have given birth before, Braxton-Hicks contractions may feel stronger this time.

Look back at the ways to tell if you're having pre-term labor contractions (Chapter 8). If contractions start to come regularly and get stronger, they may be real labor. (Learn more of the signs of real labor in Chapter 10.)

Your last prenatal visits

Your provider will want check you more often in the last few weeks of pregnancy. He is likely to check:

- How far down baby has moved and her position
- How much the cervix has changed

Your cervix starts to thin (efface) and open (dilate) in the last month. You may not feel this happening. Usually, it will change faster when you go into active labor.

The thick mucus plug from your cervix may come out with a little blood (called "bloody show").

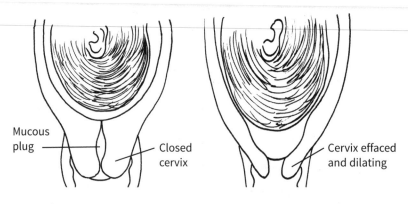

Mucous plug — Closed cervix

Cervix effaced and dilating

How your cervix opens

Effacement is the thinning of the neck of the cervix. Dilation is the opening of the hole. Both things happen as the baby's body presses down on the cervix.

Last steps to get ready

You can do many things to get yourself ready for labor.

Stay active. Continue the exercises and stretches from Chapters 3 and 8 as long as they are comfortable. Remember that squats, kegels, and massage all help you get ready for pushing. Practice tightening and relaxing.

Practice relaxing during contractions. Use your Braxton Hicks contractions to practice what you have learned about relaxing. As your belly gets hard, try the ways of breathing that you learned in birth classes.

Having sex can help you get ready for labor, too. If you want to and your provider does not say not to, you can have sex until your water breaks. You may feel contractions if you have an orgasm. Semen can also help thin the cervix. And the hormones and good feelings from sex can help you relax. See Chapter 8 for more.

Get comfortable. Standing up straight, lying on your left side, and using lots of pillows will help you in these last months. Look at the tips for getting rest earlier in this chapter. Go back to Chapter 8 for more tips on staying comfortable.

Try not to be impatient

Most babies know when it's time to be born. Once baby has reached early term (37 weeks), you don't need to worry if labor starts on its own. It means baby is likely ready to be born. Babies born in the period of 39th and 40th weeks are likely to have the best health. Baby's brain and lungs are still developing in the last few weeks. This is why it's best not to give birth too soon.

Your provider may talk about these four periods of birth:

- Early Term: weeks 37 and 38
- Full Term: weeks 39 and 40
- Late Term: 41 weeks
- Postterm: 42 weeks and beyond

If labor starts before 37 weeks, she may need extra care, but it isn't your fault. Some babies are born early no matter what you do. You still gave baby the best care possible for all the time she was inside.

Read Chapter 10

Know as much as you can about birth before it starts. You won't want to try to learn as you go, although your nurses, doctor, or midwife will be able to help you.

Know signs of labor starting

Remind yourself about what will happen and when to call your provider.

Give your other kids extra attention now

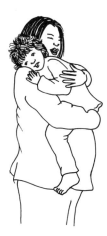

Make sure your older kids know you will have plenty of love for all of them.

Let your older kids know that you will have the baby soon. Tell them what the plan is–when you may leave, who will stay with them, and when you will be back. Think of something special they can do, either for their own fun or to welcome baby. Let them know when they will be able to see you and meet baby.

Remember, your baby can hear the sounds you make. Have your partner and other kids talk to her. She'll know your voices when she is born.

If you are planning a home birth, think about if you want your other kids there with you. You would need to tell them what to expect. The sights and sounds of labor and delivery could be scary. If they are old enough to understand, ask them if they want to be there. Talk with your midwife about how to prepare them.

It's best to have someone you trust come over to care for them even if they say they want to be with you. That way, they could change their minds, go out, have food, and play while you and your partner are busy.

Get the practical things done

☐ Register at the hospital or birth center ahead of time. This will make everything easier when you arrive in labor.

☐ Pack your bag. (See Chapter 10 for a list of things to take along.)

☐ Plan how to get to the hospital. Who will drive you? You might want to ask more than one person, in case one is busy. Does that person know how to get there?

☐ Check with friends who have said they would help after you come home. Make sure they can do it.

☐ Choose baby's doctor or nurse. Look back at Chapter 5 for tips on making this big decision.

Things to have ready at home

☐ Some cooked meals in the freezer

☐ Menstrual pads (not tampons)

☐ Diapers and other baby supplies

☐ Mild laundry soap for baby's clothes

Write down your birth plan

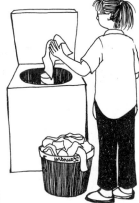

A birth plan is a list or letter about how you want your labor and birth to go. It's a tool to talk with your provider about what kind of care you want. If you give birth in a hospital, it helps the nurses, doctors, and midwives know your goals. It will also help you and your support person(s) keep track of the decisions you've made.

Ask friends and relatives to help around the house.

What to include

Make your birth plan after you have learned all about labor and birth. Talk to your childbirth class leader about what to put in it. Ask your doctor, midwife, or nurse, too. Providers are more likely to read it if it fits on one page, so think about what's most important to you.

No matter what kind of birth you end up having, you will have choices to make. Think about your perfect birth. What makes it perfect for you and for baby?

Now, think about some of the tricky things that could come up during labor and birth. What do you feel strongly about? Write those down, too. It's very hard to think clearly in labor, so having things written down is helpful.

What else?

If you are planning a home birth or birth center birth, it's a good idea to make a "plan B" birth plan for in case you end up in the hospital. Ask your provider what things you should include. (Go back to Chapter 5 to review what is different in the hospital.)

Write down any choices you've made about how you want your baby to be cared for right after birth, too.

My Birth Plan

These are my wishes. I know I can change my mind at any time.
I also know the things I want may not happen if problems come up.

Name: _____

- My birth partner/support team for labor: _____

- I want to be able to walk around during labor. Yes ___ No ___

- I want to have medication as early as possible. Yes ___ No ___

- I want no pain medication. Yes ___ No ___

- If I need medication, I'd like this kind: _____

- How will I decide I need them? _____

- I would like to try these positions during labor: (circle) standing, sitting,
  squatting, other _____.

- I do not want an episiotomy if possible. Please use other methods to avoid
  tearing or cutting. Yes ___ No ___

- I would like _____ to cut the cord.

- I want to breastfeed my baby right away. Yes ___ No ___

  I would like my baby to get breastmilk only until we go home. Yes ___ No ___

- I want my baby to stay in my room all the time. Yes ___ No ___

- In case of a c-section, I would like to to watch or have the doctor tell me what
  is happening. Yes ___ No ___ . My birth partner wants to be with me during the
  c-section. Yes ___ No ___

- If I have a baby boy, I want him to be circumcised. Yes ___ No ___

- I want medicine to be used to reduce the baby's pain. Yes ___ No ___

- I and my partner want to be present. Yes ___ No ___

- It will be a religious ceremony. Yes ___ No ___

- Other things I want my caregivers to know to know:

  _____

  _____

  _____

  _____

  _____

Be realistic about your goals

It's important to think about your goals before you're in labor. It helps everyone around you support you and your baby. When you talk to your providers, ask them what they think of your plan. Sometimes hospital rules get in the way of some goals. Sometimes you and your provider may feel very differently about something. A birth plan is also a way to let them know what you feel strongly about, are scared of, and are excited about. Some things can be argued, but your feelings can't. This can help your partner or care team work with you.

What do you do with the plan?

Ask to have it put in your chart. Bring a few copies with you to your birth. If in the hospital, ask the nurse to post it by the door or on the front of your chart.

Remember that each labor and birth is different. Things may not go the way you put in your birth plan. Or, you may change your mind about something. You birth plan is just your goals. If things change, ask questions until you feel okay about what's happening. Don't be afraid to ask your providers to explain things. If it is emergency, they won't let your questions keep them from helping you or your baby.

Tips for partners

- Be ready. Know the signs of labor. Know when to call the doctor, midwife, or nurse. Know when to go to the hospital or birth center, and how to get there.

- Watch out for warning signs for labor (page 110) and high blood pressure (page 119).

- Practice what you learned to help her relax during labor.

- Talk about the birth plan. Be sure you know what she wants and doesn't want so you can support her when it's time.

- Be patient. Your partner may be very tired and uncomfortable in these last weeks. Help her stay relaxed as you both wait for baby.

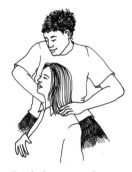

"It feels so good to have my partner rub my shoulders."

Month-to-month checkups

Month 7

Questions to ask at my seven-month checkup

- *How long should I plan to keep working?*
- *Am I likely to go into labor early (preterm labor)?*
- *Do I have inverted nipples?*
- *I eat lots of vegetables, fruit, and grains but still get constipated. What else can I do?*
- *Should I start counting how often my baby moves?*
- *If you are expecting twins: Is there anything special I should know to prevent preterm labor?*

Other questions I have:

1. _____
   _____
   _____

2. _____
   _____
   _____

3. _____
   _____
   _____

Your seven-month checkup notes

Today, _____, I had my seven-month appointment.

I am _____ weeks pregnant. I weigh _____ pounds/kg.

I have gained _____ pounds/kg since my last checkup.

My blood pressure is _____ (see below).

Things I learned today

1. _____

   _____

   _____

2. _____

   _____

   _____

My next checkup will be on

The _____ of _____, at _____:_____.
      (date)   **(month)**   **(time)**

Questions to ask at your next checkup

- *Is my baby growing well?*
- *Can my partner and I still have sex and what positions are best at this time?*
- *Is my baby head down or head up?*
- *How is my blood pressure?*
- *What kind of exercise should I do now?*
- *How do I register at the hospital or birth center before I go into labor?*

Other questions I have:

1. _____

   _____

   _____

2. _____

   _____

   _____

My eight-month checkup #1 notes

On this date, _____, I had my first eight-month appointment.
I am _____ weeks pregnant. I weigh _____ pounds/kg.
I have gained _____ pounds/kg since my last checkup.
My blood pressure is _____ (see below).
My baby's position: _____.

Things I learned today

1. _____
   _____

2. _____
   _____

3. _____
   _____

My doctor or nurse-midwife wants me to call when I have these signs of labor:

1. _____
   _____

2. _____
   _____

3. _____
   _____

4. _____
   _____

My next checkup will be on

The _____ of _____, at _____:_____.
      (date)   **(month)**   **(time)**

My eight-month checkup #2 notes

On this date, _____, I had my second eight-month appointment.

I am _____ weeks pregnant. I weigh _____ pounds/kg now.

I have gained _____ pounds/kg since my last checkup.

I have gained _____ pounds/kg since I got pregnant.

My blood pressure is _____.

Things I learned today

1. _____

   _____

2. _____

   _____

3. _____

   _____

My next checkup will be on

The _____ of _____, at _____:_____.
     (date)   (month)   (time)

Questions to ask at your nine-month checkups

- *How will I know if my contractions are real labor? When should I call you?*

- *What positions (sitting, squatting, or lying down) do you think work best during labor?*

- *If I need pain medication, what kinds would you advise? What side effects would they have for my baby and me?*

- *Who can help me with breastfeeding?*

- *Do I need a Group B Strep test?*

Other questions I have:

1. _____

   _____

2. _____

   _____

Use the last page of this chapter to write things you want to remember about this important time.

My nine-month checkup #1 notes

On this date, _____, I had my first nine-month appointment.

I weigh _____ pounds/kg now.

I have gained _____ pounds/kg since my last checkup.

My baby has dropped? Yes ___ No ___

I am _____ percent effaced and _____ centimeters dilated. (This may not be measured at every checkup this month.)

My baby's position is head down ___ or bottom down ___.

Things I learned today

1. _____

_____

2. _____

_____

3. _____

_____

My next checkup will be on

The _____ of _____, at _____:_____.
　　　(date)　　　　　(month)　　　　　　(time)

(Notes pages for the next few weekly visits are at the end of this chapter.)

My nine-month checkup #2 notes

Date _____

I weigh _____ pounds/kg now.

I have gained _____ pounds/kg since I got pregnant.

I am _____ percent effaced and _____ centimeters dilated (if measured).

Things I learned today

1. _____

   _____

2. _____

   _____

3. _____

   _____

My next checkup will be on

The _____ of _____, at _____:_____.
     (date)   **(month)**   **(time)**

My nine-month checkup #3 notes

Date _____ I weigh _____ pounds/kg now.

I am _____ percent effaced and _____ centimeters dilated (if measured).

Things I learned today

1. _____

_____

2. _____

_____

3. _____

_____

My next checkup will be on

The _____ of _____, at _____:_____.
　　　　(date)　　　　　(month)　　　　　(time)

My nine-month checkup #4 notes

Date _____ I weigh ____ pounds/kg now.

I am _____ percent effaced and _____ centimeters dilated (if measured).

Things I learned today

1. _____

_____

2. _____

_____

3. _____

_____

How I am feeling now

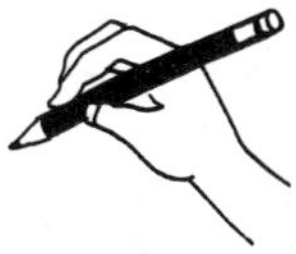

_____

_____

_____

_____

_____

_____

_____

You can keep notes on what happened during labor and delivery at the end of Chapter 10.

The big day is almost here!

Whether your pregnancy has been easy or not, you know it will end soon. You will soon have a new child to love. You have already started to be a parent by taking care of your unborn baby.

What names are you thinking of giving your baby?

_____

_____

_____

How do you feel now?

___ Excited ___ Scared ___ Happy ___ Depressed

___ A little bit of all of these

Other feelings?

_____

_____

_____

What are your special hopes?

_____

_____

_____

Do you have new concerns now?

_____

_____

_____

Share how you feel with your partner or with a close friend.

_____

_____

_____

_____

_____

_____

_____

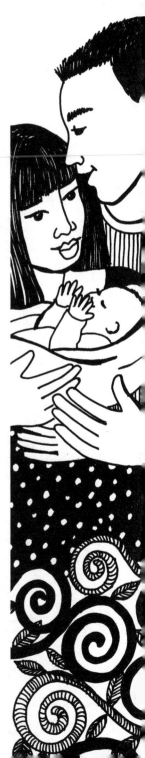

Chapter 10

Your Baby's Birth

By now, you probably feel very tired of being pregnant and ready to move on to parenthood. As you wait for your baby's birth, you likely feel both excited and worried.

Giving birth is a natural and amazing thing. It may seem strange and intense, but your body will know what to do. Learning what to expect can help you feel ready and make birth less scary.

Look in this chapter for:

How birth happens naturally, page 140

Beginning of labor, is it real?

Straight talk about pain

When to call your doctor or midwife, page 143

STAGE 1: Labor, page 144

Contractions; Tips for birth partners

Active labor; Tips for birth partners

Transition: the hardest part

STAGE 2: The birth of your baby, page 149

STAGE 3: Delivery of the placenta, page 151

STAGE 4: Beginning of recovery, page 151

Other things to know about birth, page 152

Drugs, epidural, episiotomy, c-section

Labor and Birth Surprises

Baby's Birth Day, page 162

Be ready ahead of time

This chapter will tell you all about normal birth. It also gives information about medical procedures (drugs or surgery) that you might need for a safe delivery. You will also find information on some surprises that could come along. Try to read all of it before your ninth month.

We hope you have been able to take a childbirth class. If you have not been able to go to a class, be sure to tell your provider.

Your birth plan

Remember the birth plan in Chapter 9? If you haven't done it, now is the time to do it. Reading this chapter will help you decide about your wishes. Give the plan to your provider and make sure your birth partner has a copy.

Information for the hospital or birth center

Fill this out before labor begins:

Your blood type (ask your provider) _____

Any problems with your pregnancy? (diabetes, high blood pressure, etc.) _____

_____

Your doctor or midwife_____

Phone # _____ 24-hour phone # _____

Baby's doctor or nurse _____

Phone # _____ 24-hour phone # _____

Insurance company or plan _____

Your policy # _____

Your birth partner (name and phone #)

_____

Do you have a birth plan? no ___ yes ___ (If yes, where is it?)

_____

Your contacts in an emergency: (names and phone numbers)

_____

_____

What should I take with me?

Pack most of these things ahead of time. Check off each thing as you pack it.

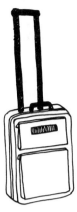

__ Your ID and insurance card

__ Your birth plan

__ This book

__ A watch with a second hand or a smart phone with a timer for timing contractions.

__ A pen and paper for notes.

__ A way to play your favorite music. Soft, quiet music can help you relax during labor.

__ A camera with a full battery and the charger.

__ Your phone charger

__ Sugar-free candy to keep your mouth moist.

__ Clothes or a nightgown to wear if you don't want to use a hospital gown. Take a short robe or sweater that opens in front, slippers, and warm socks.

__ Hairbrush, hair ties, toothbrush and toothpaste. Prescription medicines.

__ Other things that may help you feel fresh, like face wash, deodorant, lotion, or makeup.

__ Money for your birth partner(s) to buy coffee and food.

__ Snacks to help keep you both going. Dried fruit, nut butter, and cheese or yogurt can give you energy.

__ A nursing bra.

__ Stretchy or loose clothes to wear home.

__ Clothes for baby to wear home: an outfit with legs, socks, and a hat (Gowns and skirts don't let the car seat harness fit safely.)

__ A few thin baby blankets and one thick one.

__ Car seat for the ride home. You and your baby must ride buckled up, even in a taxi. If you do not have a car seat, ask if the hospital sells low-cost seats.

How Birth Happens Naturally

This part of the chapter follows the flow of the birth process. Find notes for birth partners with each stage of childbirth.

The main event

No one can say for sure when your labor will start, but you can be sure it will happen soon. Some people have clear signs before it begins. Others do not.

In the last few weeks before the birth, your baby drops (moves down) between the pelvic bones. You may see your belly is lower. Your cervix softens, thins, and starts to opens. (See pictures, Chapter 9, page 122.) Now your real contractions will begin.

Labor usually starts any time from two weeks before your due date to two weeks after. Labor may last a few hours or more than a day. Labor often will take longer the first time than with second or third babies.

Try to be patient. A baby's body needs at least 39 weeks in the uterus. His brain, lungs, and liver are still growing. Babies born too soon do not have fat to stay warm. They also may not be able to see or hear as well.

Beginnings of labor

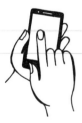

There are a number of signs of labor. You may not have all of them. Ask your doctor or midwife what else to watch for.

- A glob of thick mucus (called the mucus plug) with a little bright red blood that comes out of your vagina.
- Clear fluid that gushes or leaks from your vagina. This is the bag of waters (amniotic sac) breaking. This may happen before or after contractions start.
- Low back pain that will not go away or low belly cramps (like when you have your period).
- Very soft bowel movements (or diarrhea).
- Contractions that get stronger, last longer, and come closer and closer together.

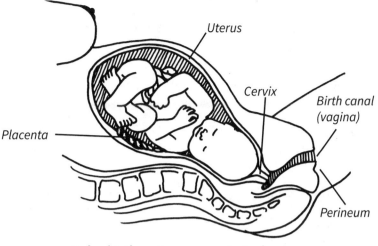

Uterus

Cervix

Birth canal (vagina)

Placenta

Perineum

Baby in the uterus—parts to know

Call any time, day or night. It is better to call early than to wait too long. You may be asked to stay at home for a while, or to take a walk close by. If your water has broken, your provider will likely want to see you within a few hours.

Ask her when you should go to the hospital or birth center. If you are planning a home birth, ask when she will come over.

Is it real labor?

It can be hard to tell if your contractions are real. You've felt contractions on and off in the last months. Try these things:

- Lie down and rest for a while.
- Get up and walk around.
- Drink a big glass of water and have a small snack.

If doing these things make the contractions stop or get weaker or slower, you're probably not really in labor. Real labor contractions don't stop coming once they start.

Time your contractions (see pages 146–147 on how to time). Early contractions are about a half-minute long and come about every 15 to 30 minutes.

If you are not sure, call your doctor or midwife. She will not mind being called at any time. Sometimes the only way to know if true labor has started is to be checked by your provider. She can feel where baby is and how much your cervix has changed.

The Basic Stages of Labor

1st Stage: Labor (Opening of the cervix)

The cervix opens (dilates) and thins (effaces) to let the baby through. Contractions become stronger and faster as the uterus pushes baby down into the cervix. This is the longest stage of childbirth.

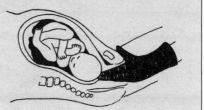

2nd Stage: Birth of your baby (Delivery)

With your help, the uterus contractions push baby through the open cervix, into the vagina. The vagina and perineum stretch wide open and the baby comes out.

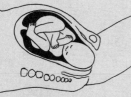
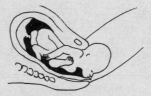
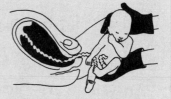

In the second stage, the baby is first pushed all the way down the birth canal.

Next, the baby's head comes through the opening.

Last, the baby's body comes out. Baby begins to breathe on its own.

3rd Stage: Delivery of the placenta

The placenta comes off the wall of the uterus. The uterus contracts to push it out through the vagina. This stage is much less painful. Baby may be put on your chest during this stage and for recovery.

4th Stage: Recovery

The uterus starts to shrink while you rest and relax. This is a good time to breastfeed and talk to your baby. Baby will be examined and wrapped up. All this can be done while baby is on your chest. You will get stitches if you have a tear or cut in your perineum.

When to Call Your Doctor or Midwife

Ask your provider when she wants you to call. Write down what she says:

_____

_____

When in doubt, call if:

- ◆ Your bag of waters breaks.
- ◆ Your contractions have been 5 to 10 minutes apart for at least an hour.
- ◆ You cannot walk or talk during contractions.

Tell your provider as much as you can about what is going on. When you can't talk, ask your partner to talk to her.

Straight talk about pain

Pain will be a natural part of your birth. There is no need to be scared. It comes from the work your body is doing.

Normal pain comes from the contractions of the uterus, the widening of the birth canal and pelvis, the stretching of the perineum. Stress, pain, and contractions all make the body release natural pain control (endorphins). This can be very powerful.

Labor pain often starts as a dull back ache or cramps that come and go. The cramping gets much stronger as contractions come closer together and last longer. As you start to push, the stretching of your pelvis, vagina, and perineum will hurt. Once baby is out, almost all of the pain is gone right away. Then, your baby can help distract you from the rest.

Giving birth without drugs can make you feel very good and very strong. If your labor is going well, you may only need some relaxation and comfort methods to get you through it.

How to have less pain naturally

- ◆ Have a birth partner and/or a doula to support, comfort, and encourage you.
- ◆ Use breathing and massage methods to relax.
- ◆ Change positions—sit up, squat, kneel, get on hands and knees, sit on a birth ball, rock in a rocker.

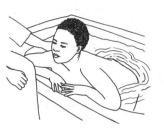

- Walk slowly as your partner holds you.
- Sit in a shower or soak in a warm (not hot) tub—after you are at least 6 cm dilated.
- Focus on the important job you are doing and know it won't last much longer.

Help for back pain

Contractions can make your back tired and sore. This pain can be very strong if baby is facing your front. (Most babies face the back during labor.) When baby faces front, his head pushes hard on your bones, which can hurt a lot. Try the comfort methods above. Here are other things that can help:

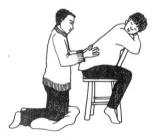

- Have your partner push firmly on your low back.
- Put a heat pad or cold pack on your low back.
- Let your partner massage your back and hips.
- Lean forward against your partner, a table or bed, or on a birth ball. Or rest your head on a pillow while you kneel on a bed or the ground. These poses take the strain off of your back and let baby hang down.

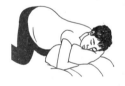

- Lie on your side if you get in bed. Try and rest.
- Get in the shower and have your partner spray the water on your low back. Close your eyes and relax.

These things can help a lot. But, if labor is very long or contractions are very hard, you may need more help. Pain makes you very tired. If you are too tired or hurting too much, pain medicines can help. Using them doesn't mean you have failed in any way.

For details about drugs used for pain, see the section on drugs and surgery later in this chapter (pages 152–158).

STAGE 1: Labor

During pregnancy, the uterus has grown into the largest, strongest muscle in your body. When labor starts, it contracts without any help from you. This can feel very strange at first.

Your job is to help the uterus by letting it do its work. Relax as much as you can during contractions and rest in between. Move around, like walking or trying different positions. Stay upright by standing, sitting, squatting, or kneeling. Just lying down in bed can slow labor.

Let contractions do the work

In labor, your uterus is working to open the cervix. Your cervix stretches from tightly closed to wide open, 10 cm (centimeters) or 4 inches, during this stage.

There are three parts of labor. Your body has to work harder and harder as the cervix opens more.

- **Early labor:** Contractions are short and not very strong. Your cervix opens to 4 centimeters. You can usually stay at home during this time. Being where you're relaxed and comfortable will help early labor go faster.

- **Active labor:** Contractions are longer and stronger. They come closer together. Your cervix will open to 8 centimeters. You should go to the birth center or hospital now. For a home birth, you should call your midwife to your house now if you haven't already.

- **Transition:** The cervix widens completely, from 8 to 10 centimeters. It might have to stretch a bit more if baby's head is very big.

Imagine your baby's head pushing through the opening of a turtleneck shirt.

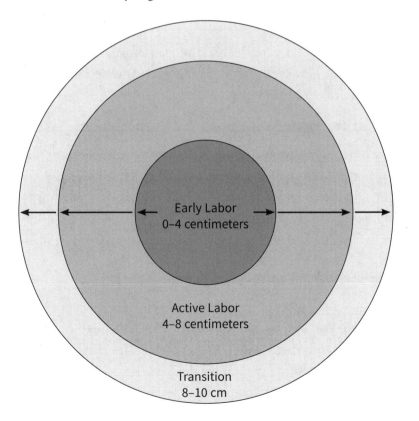

Early Labor
0–4 centimeters

Active Labor
4–8 centimeters

Transition
8–10 cm

The real size of your cervix as it stretches around your baby's head!

Contractions in this part are the hardest, strongest, and closest together. You may not have time to rest much between them. Try not to push just yet. Pushing too soon can slow the opening of the cervix. Your provider can tell you when it's safe to push.

More about early labor

Early labor can take a few hours or a few days. You will be more comfortable at home at this time. There is no need to be in the hospital or birth center until you are in active labor. Getting to the hospital early does not help your baby come quicker and you may be sent home.

Go back to pages 141 and 143 for signs of labor and when to call your doctor or midwife. Also, call if you or the baby suddenly feel different or if you have questions.

While you are in early labor, you can do some normal things, like cook, take a walk, watch a move, and visit with friends. Eat lightly and drink water or juice. Try to relax and take naps, but don't just lie down the whole time. Sitting up, standing, and walking help the baby move down into the birth canal. Let gravity help pull baby down.

During a contraction, try the breathing and relaxation exercises you have learned. Have your partner time your contractions so you know when to call your provider.

Tips for birth partners: Keep track of contractions

 Knowing how long, strong, and far apart your contractions are is an important role for a birth partner. This will tell both of you and your provider how labor is going. Use a timer or a watch with a second hand to time contractions. Put the information into the form in the box on the next page.

Active labor: When mom's work really starts

Once you are checked in to the hospital, a labor and delivery nurse will help you know what to do. If you go to a birth center or are at home, your midwife will help guide you. These nurses and midwives have helped many families in labor. They will have a lot of tips for you and your partner or birth team. Their advice about

Hey, birth partners! Time to time contractions

Write the exact time when each contraction starts and stops. Figure out how long they last and how far apart they are (from start time to start time).

Note other things that happen, such as her bag of waters breaking.

Start time	Stop time	How long was it?	How far apart?	Other Signs*
_____	_____	_____	_____	_____
_____	_____	_____	_____	_____
_____	_____	_____	_____	_____
_____	_____	_____	_____	_____
_____	_____	_____	_____	_____
_____	_____	_____	_____	_____

(Use another piece of paper to continue your notes.)

Use this chart below to see what phase of labor mom is in

Phase	how long (seconds)	how often* (minutes)	centimeters dilated
Early labor	30–45 seconds	15–30 minutes	0–4 cm
Active labor	45–60 seconds	3–5 minutes	4–8 cm
Transition	45–90 seconds	2–3 minutes	8–10 cm

*Count how many minutes pass from the start of one contraction to the start of the next one.

positions, what to do, and how to breathe can be very helpful. If you have a doctor, she will likely check in on you from time to time. She'll likely come back and stay when you start to push. Until then, nurses will be with you to help.

Stay comfortable

Staying calm and relaxed helps labor go more smoothly and hurt less. Make sure the nurses or your midwife have your birth plan.

Drink water or juice or suck on ice chips to stay hydrated. Go to the bathroom as you need to. Many women find sitting on the toilet very comfortable in labor.

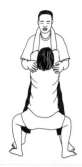

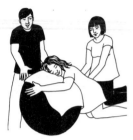

Two comfortable positions

It will be easier to relax in a quiet, peaceful room. Play music that you like. Post a "quiet" sign on the door or ask people to wait outside if you feel the need.

Most mothers do not go through labor lying down. Moving around and being upright can be more comfortable and help labor move along.

Some positions to try:

◆ Walk or slow-dance with your partner.

◆ Stand and lean back or forward into your partner.

◆ Rest on your hands and knees.

◆ Fold your arms on a birth ball while kneeling.

◆ Squat and lean back or forward into your partner.

If active labor goes on for a long time, gets too painful for you, or you start to feel too tired to go on, you may want to ask for some pain medicine.

Tips for birth partners: During active labor

Your biggest job is to help your partner relax during contractions and stay comfortable. You could:

◆ Keep timing the contractions.

◆ Help mom change positions, massaging her back.

◆ Give support when she walks to the bathroom or around the room.

◆ Offer ice chips or foods that are okay to have.

◆ Help with the relaxation methods you both learned in class.

You are mom's protector. Key ways to do this:

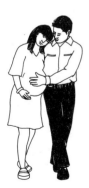

◆ Keep the room quiet so she can concentrate or play music she wants; ask chatty visitors to talk somewhere else.

◆ Make sure the nurses or midwife have the birth plan. If you notice the plan isn't being followed, ask that person to explain.

◆ Speak up if you think your partner is having problems. Ask the labor nurse to check that all is okay.

◆ Keep yourself strong by taking breaks and eating when you need to.

Transition: Stretching the cervix completely open

This is the last part of labor, when your cervix opens the last two centimeters. This is the hardest part and can be very painful and tiring.

Your contractions will be very strong. You may feel like you have no break between them. Many women can't talk or pay attention to anything other than their body now.

Your provider will check your cervix to make sure it's all the way open before telling you to start pushing. Pushing before your cervix is ready can make it stop opening. If your body feels like pushing before the cervix is all the way open, try to breathe to relax and wait.

STAGE 2: The birth of your baby!

Once your cervix is all the way open, you can start pushing your baby through the birth canal. You will likely feel the need to push during contractions. This may feel like you need to have a bowel movement (poop).

Try not to hold your breath while pushing. Take a few quick breaths as you push. Then rest until the next contraction starts.

This stage can take some time. Your midwife or nurse will be with you. She will check on how far down the baby has moved. Every push helps stretch your vagina to move baby down the birth canal. Help him along by spending some time walking, sitting, or squatting. These positions allow gravity to help. You can give birth lying on your back, but gravity won't be able to help.

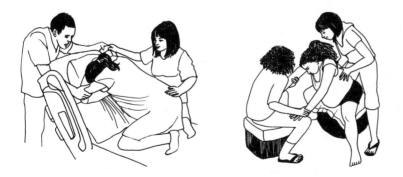 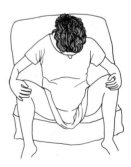

Three positions that are good for pushing in Stage 2

Sometimes, your doctor or midwife may ask you not to push during a contraction. When you aren't pushing, she can check on baby's cord. This also gives time for the perineum to stretch. Panting or low moaning can help you keep from pushing.

When the baby's head is all the way down in your vagina, your provider can see it. Your perineum must stretch wide enough for it. The skin may burn or sting.

Ways your provider can help baby come through the perineum more easily include:

- Slowing down delivery a little by pressing her hand on baby's head.

- Using a warm cloth or gentle massage to help avoid tearing.

- Making a cut in the perineum to widen the opening (an episiotomy). (See page 155.)

Even if the opening is wide enough, sometimes a baby's head won't come out as it should. The provider may use forceps or a vacuum extractor to keep baby from slipping back in between pushes. This will guide his head out.

Once your baby's head and shoulders are out, the rest of his body slips out quickly. You will feel great relief and have much less pain.

When baby first comes out, she may be very still and quiet. The doctor or midwife may need to clear her nose and mouth to help her take her first breath. Then she will probably start to cry as her lungs fill with air for the first time.

If you ask, your provider probably will put baby right on your chest or belly. It is good for you and baby to have him on your bare chest for the first hour or so. Finally, you can hold the baby you worked so hard for!

Cutting the cord

After birth, your provider will clamp and cut the cord. Cutting the cord does not hurt you or your baby. Your partner may want to cut the cord.

You may want to ask your provider to wait until the cord stops pulsing to clamp the cord. This lets all of baby's blood drain from the placenta into his body. This can help give baby a healthy start.

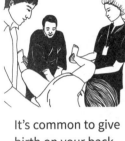

It's common to give birth on your back. But being more upright is often an easier way for baby to be born.

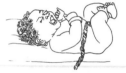

Cord blood can be saved for use in research or for curing some rare diseases. If you want to do this, the American Academy of Pediatrics advises donating it to a public cord-blood bank.

Tips for birth partners: During Stage 2

- Helping mom get into positions to help baby come out.
- Wiping her forehead and cheeks with a cool washcloth.
- Being positive about how she's doing; staying calm if she moans and cries.
- Reminding her that she's almost done, telling her when baby's head begins to show.
- Staying fairly quiet, so mom can focus and can hear what her provider is telling her.
- Cutting the cord if you want to.

STAGE 3: Delivery of the placenta

In a few more minutes, the placenta will come off the wall of your uterus. Contractions will continue to push it out, but they will be much more gentle. You may not even feel them. Or your provider may ask you to push a few more times.

Your provider will check to make sure all of it has come out. Your nurse or midwife may rub your belly firmly to help your tired uterus. You may get some medicine to help it stop bleeding.

Tips for birth partners: When the hard part is over

- Ask the nurse to bring a warm blanket, and get mom a snack and a drink if she wants one.
- Ask the nurse to wait before giving baby a bath so you both can enjoy him first.

STAGE 4: Beginning of recovery

The hard part is over! You did it! Now your nurse or midwife will help you get cleaned up and comfortable.

If you had an episiotomy or tear, your doctor or midwife will stitch it up. This can take a few minutes. She will numb the area so you don't feel it.

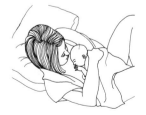

Now you can relax. You can cuddle and nurse your baby. Drink some water or juice, eat, and rest.

Your uterus should start shrinking right away. You may feel more contractions. Your nurse or midwife will feel your belly to check its size. She may massage your uterus to help it contract. You may be able to feel it yourself. Reach down and press on your lower belly. Your uterus should feel hard and be about the size of a grapefruit.

You will have bleeding from your vagina for at least a few weeks. This means you will need to wear large pads.

This is a perfect time to breastfeed. New babies are usually awake and eager to feed in the first hour after birth. Your baby will know the smell of your breast milk. It smells like the amniotic fluid on her body. If she's not hungry, let her lie on your chest with her head near your breast.

Tips for partners: Help with recovery

- Enjoy this time with mom and your new baby.
- Help with breastfeeding.
- Try kangaroo care for the first time when baby isn't nursing. Open your shirt and cuddle baby on your bare chest. Put a warm blanket over both of you.
- Get mom a face cloth and towel so she can wash her face.

Other Things to Know About Birth

Drugs or surgery you may need

Of course, sometimes birth needs some medical help along the way. These are often called "interventions" or "procedures." Learn about them before you go into labor. If your provider thinks you need an intervention, you will want to know what it is. That will help you to ask why it is needed and give your consent.

If your provider advises doing one of these things, make sure you understand what it is. Unless there is an emergency, you will be asked if you agree (give consent). Questions to ask:

- *How will this drug or surgery help me?*
- *How quickly do we have to decide?*
- *What are the benefits and risks to me?*
- *Are there any other ways that might be less risky?*

When labor doesn't start on its own

Labor can be started (induced) using drugs or other ways to get the cervix to open and contractions to start. It is usually best to wait for your body to start labor naturally. This is why most providers do not want to start labor early "just to get it over with."

But, there are some important medical reasons to try to start labor. A common reason is if a baby is late. Late means two weeks after his due date (42 weeks). Until then, most babies are safest in their mom's belly. After 42 weeks, there is more chance of problems for mom and baby.

If baby is overdue, your doctor or midwife will likely check your cervix often to see if it is opening. To get labor started she might:

- Advise you to be active at home like walk a lot, climb stairs, have sex. Playing with your nipples can help.
- Break the bag of water ("sweep your membranes").
- Give you a drug like Pitocin. Sometimes this works fast, but it can take a long time.

Women who have labor induced have a higher chance of needing a c-section. Your provider may feel it is worth this risk if you or your baby have medical problems. These might be an infection, your bag of waters is low on fluid, you or baby has blood pressure problems or baby has stopped growing as he should.

Drugs to help with pain

Giving birth is hard work and drugs have limits. There is no way to make birth painless. Pain medicines (drugs) can help with some of the pain, but not all of it.

It is good to learn how to manage pain and to practice ways to relax. Labor tends to go faster if you wait as long as you can before taking a drug. So, even if you want pain medicine, you will still need to cope with some pain in the earlier parts of labor. Also, drugs don't always work as quickly or as well as you want them to.

Kinds of pain medication

Learn about what kinds of pain relief there are, when they can be used, and their side effects. At a prenatal checkup, ask your provider what kinds of drugs she prefers to use and why. Tell your partner and provider what you would like to use and put it in your birth plan.

Different kinds of drugs are used depending on:

◆ How you are doing.

◆ How baby is doing.

◆ What progress you have made in labor.

These drugs usually are very safe, but may have some side effects. It is important to know the risks before you agree to use any drug. Ask your provider about the side effects before labor starts. Think about your options now, since it's hard to make decisions when you're in labor.

◆ **Pain drugs** are narcotics. You feel less pain but still feel the peak of each contraction and the urge to push. Pain drugs cannot be used in the pushing stage because they may affect baby's breathing. They might make you feel dizzy, itchy, or like throwing up.

◆ **Sleep aids** may help you rest in the early stage of labor. They may help you relax if you are nervous or tired. They may be given with narcotics. These drugs may affect your baby as well as you.

Epidural or spinal block to numb belly and legs

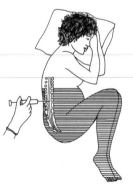

An epidural or spinal block make the lower part of your body numb so it doesn't feel pain (see picture). For a spinal block, drugs are put into your lower back with a needle. For an epidural, a large needle is used to place a very narrow tube into the space around your spinal cord in your lower back. Drugs are given through this tube. You will feel little to no pain or urge to push.

An epidural numbs the shaded area of your body.

Once you are numb, you won't be able to walk around, change positions yourself, or take a warm bath. You will be able to push during the delivery stage, but you won't feel the contractions. Your provider or a nurse will feel your uterus. When it gets hard, she will tell you to push.

In some cases, an epidural or spinal block makes labor go quicker. In other cases, it slows labor down. It may make a c-section more likely. Also, there can be side effects for mom afterwards, such as severe headache. It is, however, good to know that the drugs used have fewer effects on the newborn than other kinds of drugs.

Episiotomy—A cut through your perineum

Pushing baby through the skin around your vagina is hard work. A cut or episiotomy (ep-easy-oto-me) can be done to make a bigger opening for baby to come through.

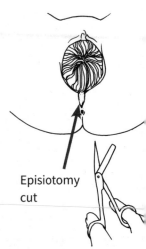

Episiotomy cut

Most women do not need episiotomies, but many providers do them often. In most births, the perineum will stretch on its own, but this takes time. Some providers want to do it to speed things up. Many women don't want to be cut because they:

- Don't want to be sore for days after birth.
- Don't want to have to care for the cut and stitches.
- Have learned that a tear often heals faster.
- Worry about other health problems it could cause later.

If you do not want an episiotomy, tell your provider and put that in your birth plan. Ask your birth partner to remind your provider during stage 2.

If there are problems as the baby is coming out, you might need an episiotomy. Ask your provider if she thinks it is really needed. If it is, she will make the area numb so you do not feel the cut or the stitches afterward.

It is hard to prevent tearing during pushing. But, these things may help:

- Push in positions that open your pelvis, such as squatting or kneeling.
- Ask your provider to put a warm wet cloth on the area during pushing.
- Try to relax and slow down your pushes when your provider tells you to.

What are forceps and vacuum extractors?

These are tools that can be used to hold onto the baby's head during delivery. Forceps are metal tongs and a vacuum extractor is a suction cup. When one is attached, then the provider can pull while you push during contractions.

One of these tools may be tried if mom is too tired to push hard enough or baby's head is stuck in the pelvis. There are some risks, but it may be needed to get baby to come out. If this does not work, then a c-section would have to be done.

Cesarean section—Surgical birth

A cesarean section is surgery to take out the baby. The doctor must cut through your belly and into your uterus. It is a major surgery that can be more risky for the mom than a vaginal birth.

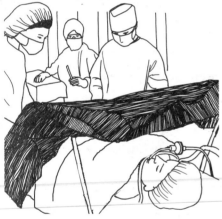

Cesareans have always been done in emergencies to save a mom's or baby's life. But, c-sections are very common now, even when there's no emergency. This is not a good thing for mom or baby. It has a small chance of very serious problems. (See risks on the next page.)

Cesarean section to take baby out using surgery.

What happens in this surgery?

You would be taken to an operating room with lots of doctors, nurses, and machines. If you have already been given a spinal or epidural, you will be awake but should feel no pain. They will make sure you are numb before they start. You may feel pulling or tugging but it won't hurt. You will not see what is happening unless you ask to. Your partner can often be in the operating room once it is time to pull baby out.

In an emergency, you may be given drugs that put you to sleep during the surgery. If this happens, your partner would be asked to wait outside.

Doctor and nurses doing a c-section.

The surgery usually takes less than 10 minutes to get the baby out. It can take up to half an hour to sew your uterus and belly back up. Your baby may be given to you or your partner to hold at this time. Sometimes baby is taken to another room while you recover or while he gets some extra help after birth. Be sure to tell the doctor if you want to hold your baby right away.

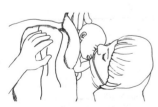

You can ask to hold baby and even breastfeed right after surgery.

You will usually stay in the hospital a day or two longer than if you had a vaginal birth. Healing at home will take much longer. You will be given medicine after the birth and to take at home, to help with the pain as you heal.

Reasons for a cesarean birth

A c-section may be needed if you or your baby has a problem that makes vaginal birth unsafe or not possible. Sometimes it is planned ahead of time. This might be the case with a breech baby (baby isn't head down), more than one baby, or if you have had a c-section before (see VBAC on page 158).

A provider may also decide that a c-section is needed if problems may have come up during labor or birth. Some of these problems are:

- Very high blood pressure (preeclampsia) in mom.
- Herpes sores in mom's vaginal area at birth.
- Baby is breech (bottom down) and cannot be turned.
- Active labor that has stopped and cannot be started again.
- Baby's position or size that makes vaginal birth impossible.
- Bad position of the umbilical cord or placenta.
- Mom or baby have a problem that makes a c-section safer.

Risks of a cesarean birth

You should know the possible risks before you choose or agree to have one. Some serious problems that a c-section could cause for a woman are:

- A bad reaction to anesthesia drugs.
- Injury to your bladder or bowel.
- A blood clot that could damage your heart or lungs.
- Wound infection.
- Death (very rare but about twice as likely compared to a vaginal birth).

Possible problems for a baby due to c-section:

- A hard time starting to breastfeed.
- Breathing problems at birth.
- Needing special care in the NICU after birth.
- Asthma or allergies in the future.
- Death (rare).

Elective cesarean birth—Not a good plan

Some women want to have a surgical birth without a medical reason. This is called elective c-section. They may be afraid of labor or want the birth to happen on a certain day. Major health agencies do not recommend this except in very special cases.

A baby should not be born early by c-section unless there is a health reason for mom or baby. Baby should stay in the uterus until at least 39 weeks, if possible.

When you didn't want a cesarean birth

If you wanted a vaginal birth but end up needing surgery, you may have a lot of mixed feelings. You might be glad that your baby is here safely, but you might be sad that your plans changed. This is normal.

If your baby needs to be born by c-section, there are some things in your birth plan you still can do. Some moms want to hear music they have chosen during or after the surgery. Some want to see the birth or have pictures taken. You may want your partner to tell you the sex of the baby and to cut the cord. You may want baby put on your chest right away to let him nurse. Many of these things can still happen if you ask. Tell your provider what is important to you.

Vaginal birth after cesarean (VBAC)

Many moms want to have a vaginal birth with their next child. They may not want to go through the hard recovery that comes after surgery. Or, they may just want to feel what it's like to have a vaginal birth. For most moms, VBAC can be safe.

Some people worry that in the next birth, the uterus will tear where it was cut for the cesarean section. This is called a uterine rupture and it is very rare. Even with this very small risk, a VBAC is likely safer than having another c-section for most women.

If you want to have a VBAC, talk to your doctor or midwife. Talk about the risks of a VBAC. Talk about the risk of another c-section. If you have a VBAC, your provider will watch closely during your labor. If there is any sign that you or baby is in danger, they may suggest another cesarean section. Most women who try to have a VBAC are able to. If your provider doesn't think a VBAC is a good idea, you can ask another one to see if they agree.

Labor and birth surprises

What if baby's head is not down?

Some babies start labor lying with head forward, head up, or sideward. Sometimes it is possible for baby to flip over during labor. Your provider may try to get baby to move by pressing on the outside of your belly. You can try getting down on hands and knees or into another position that makes space for baby to turn.

If these things do not work, your provider will check to see if baby will fit through your pelvis. Babies can be born safely bottom-first, but it may take more time and have some risks. Other positions are more risky. A c-section may be needed.

What if baby comes very fast?

Sometimes a baby might start to come out before you can get to the hospital or birth center. This is more likely if it is not your first baby. If you feel like you want to push or there's something in your vagina, call 911 right away.

> This guide does not replace help from paramedics or instructions from a health care provider by phone.

If your baby starts to come out before you get to the hospital:

1. Call 911 right away. Medics know how to deliver babies.

2. Do what the person on the phone tells you to do until helps gets there. (You also could call your doctor or midwife so they know what's happening.)

3. Do not try to drive to the hospital. If you are in the car, stop in a safe place. Lean your seat back or lie on the back seat. Put a clean cloth under your bottom.

4. If baby comes out before medics arrives, wipe his face and dry his head. Do not pull on the cord or cut it.

5. Keep baby dry and warm. Lay him on your chest against your skin. Dry baby's body. Rub him to help him breathe. Cover both of you with a blanket, coat, or sweater. Cover baby's head to keep him warm.

6. Push out the placenta. Keep it for the doctor to see.

7. Breastfeed your baby.

8. Get medical help as soon as possible.

What if your birth doesn't go as planned?

Many women spend a lot of time thinking about what their birth will be like and how they want it to go. You may have felt strongly about letting labor start on its own, not using pain medicine, or having a vaginal birth. If any of these things don't happen the way you planned, you may feel very sad, let down, or even mad.

These feelings are normal. It is important that you and your baby are healthy, but that doesn't make the other feelings go away. Some women feel like they failed or think their body is broken. These feelings can be very hard to talk about. They can make you feel guilty. Remember, it's okay and normal to feel disappointed. It doesn't mean you don't love your baby.

Share your feelings with someone who understands. Find a support group or a counselor. It is very helpful to be with other parents who have felt how you feel. Write your feelings down. It helps to work through your feelings so you can heal. Then you can focus on being a great parent to your beautiful baby.

What if baby is early?

A baby born in the 37th or 38th week is called early term. Early term babies usually do well after birth, but may need some extra care at first. This is why most babies should not be born until at least 39 weeks.

A baby born earlier than 37 weeks is called preterm or premature (a "preemie"). Twins and multiple babies often come early. Some preemies just need time to grow bigger. Others needs lots of extra care so they can grow like they would have in the uterus. Many tiny babies grow up healthy and live long lives.

*NICU is pronounced "nick-you."

A preemie who needs a lot of care would be taken to a special care nursery (newborn intensive care unit or NICU*). He would be kept in a special box (incubator or isolette) to keep warm. This might be at another hospital.

If this happens, try to spend as much time there as you can. Your baby needs to hear your voice and feel your touch even if he is very tiny. When possible, try to hold him against your skin, called kangaroo care (Chapter 11).

Get help using a breast pump so you can get your milk flowing. You will be able to bring your milk to the NICU for him when he's well enough to have it in a bottle. (See Chapter 11 for more about preemies.)

What if baby is very small even if he's not early?

Some babies born after 37 weeks are smaller than normal, under 5½ pounds (2500 grams).

A baby may be small because he has some health problems. He often needs extra special care, like a preemie. With good care, most will get healthy and live long lives.

My Baby's Birth Day!

My baby's name is_____

Baby was born on _____ at _____
                        DATE   AM / PM

Weight: _____pounds/kg   Length: _____inches

Head size (how big around): _____inches

First sign of labor:_____

_____

I got to the hospital/birth center on _____ at _____
                                       DATE   AM / PM

I was in labor for _____hours.

Things I did that helped labor go well_____

_____

_____

My birth partner(s) helped by: _____

_____

My nurses, doctor, or midwife helped by:_____

_____

Pain medicine I was given, if any_____

How I felt right after birth _____

_____

_____

Notes from my birth partner _____

_____

_____

Notes from my doctor or midwife _____

_____

_____

_____

_____

Chapter 11

Caring for Your New Baby

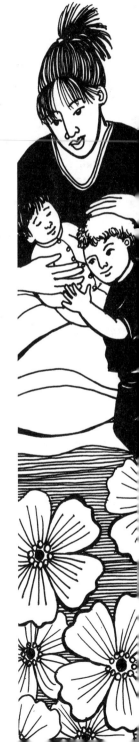

Now your baby is born. You can finally see and hold her. What an exciting time!

Once your baby begins to breathe, she is living independently. She is no longer protected by the uterus. Loud noises and bright lights are new, and the cooler air of the room could be a shock. Snuggling her against your skin is a good way to help her feel at home. Letting her breastfeed will give you both a feeling of closeness.

This and the following chapters will cover the basics.

Chapter 12—Details about feeding your baby

Chapter 13—Getting to know your baby

Chapter 14—Keeping your baby safe

Chapter 15—Keeping your baby healthy; Warning signs

Look in this chapter for:

Your new baby's health, page 164

The first day, page 166

    Feeding and holding baby

    Keeping her warm, clean, safe

    Signs of health problems to know

The first weeks at home, page 172

    Holding and carrying your baby

    Changing diapers, bathing baby

If your baby needs special care, page 178

Tips for partners, page 179

Your new baby's health

Your provider will look at your baby to make sure she is doing well. Most of these checks can be done with baby on your chest or nursing. In the first few minutes after birth, your provider will check:

- ◆ heart rate
- ◆ breathing and skin color
- ◆ temperature
- ◆ muscles and reflexes
- ◆ weight and length

Soon after, your provider will:

Hold baby when she's getting shots or getting blood taken. Cuddling may help her feel less pain.

The eye medicine can make her eyesight fuzzy for a while. You can ask to have the medicine put in after you have had time together.

- ◆ Give baby a shot of vitamin K to prevent bleeding problems.
- ◆ Put medicine in her eyes to prevent infection.
- ◆ Draw some blood from baby's heel for a "newborn screen." The blood will be tested to check for some rare but very serious problems. Often a second screen is done after a week. This is important to catch any problems that might have been missed the first time.
- ◆ Take blood for a jaundice (bilirubin) screening.
- ◆ Test baby for heart problems.
- ◆ Check baby's hearing.

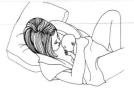

It is good for baby to hold her on your bare skin. As you hold her, you will both be covered up to stay warm. The nurse or midwife may offer to help clean baby up and put a diaper and hat on her. If all is well, you can hold her and breastfeed her as long as you want. She doesn't need a bath right away. The white vernix helps her skin stay healthy.

Welcome your baby

Many newborn babies are wide awake for a few hours after birth and then take a long nap. When baby sleeps, you should try to nap too.

After birth you may feel very emotional. Some parents feel great love for their babies right away. Others can't believe the birth has really happened. Some are too tired or sore to be able to

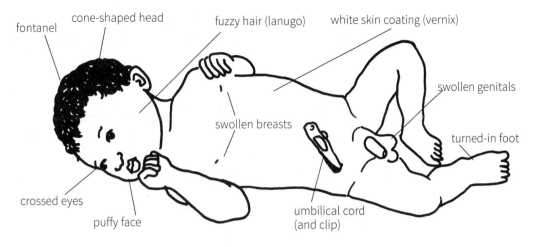

fontanel — cone-shaped head — fuzzy hair (lanugo) — white skin coating (vernix)

swollen genitals

swollen breasts

turned-in foot

crossed eyes

puffy face

umbilical cord
(and clip)

What a newborn baby looks like

focus on baby. Many parents look at their brand new baby and
wonder how they will be able to take care of such a tiny person.
All of these feelings are normal right now. You will all feel better
after you get some rest.

What your newborn looks like

A baby who has just been born looks very different from a baby
who is even a month old. A newborn will change a lot in the first
few weeks.

Your baby's face may seem puffy. Her eyes may be swollen and
may not look in the same direction. If you had a vaginal delivery,
her head is likely to be cone-shaped and her nose flattened. This is
from being squeezed coming through the birth canal. All of these
things are normal and should go away.

Your baby's skin may have a reddish color, with little white
spots (milia) on her nose, cheeks, and chin. The creamy white
coating (vernix) on her skin at birth may stay in the folds of her
skin. She may have fine, soft hair in her back and face (lanugo).
Her skin may be dry and peeling. One foot may be turned in. Her
hands and feet may look blue or purple and feel cool. All of these
things are normal and should get better soon. Lots of babies are
born with red, brown, or even blue or gray birth marks. Scratches
or bruises from birth will heal.

Her head will have two soft spots called fontanels. These are places where the bones of her skull have not grown together yet. If you press gently, you can feel a large one on the top and a small one on the back. The fontanels will close slowly by about 18 months of age. A strong layer under the skin protects her brain.

Amazing things a new baby can do

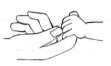

Your new baby can see things close to her. She can see your face when you hold her. She can hear and likes calm, soft, high voices. She can taste and smell.

Your baby's body moves on its own in some ways. These are called reflexes. These will go away in a few weeks or months. Watch for these reflexes now:

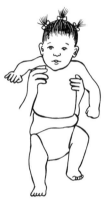

- When you touch the palm of her hand, she will hold your finger tightly.
- If you stroke her cheek, she will turn her head and open her mouth (rooting).
- When she hears a loud sound, she will startle (jerk suddenly).
- If you hold her up with her feet touching a table, she will lift up one foot (like stepping).

Example of a reflex: When her feet touch something, she will lift one foot.

The first day

New baby care is very basic: keep your baby warm, fed, comforted, and clean. The nurse, midwife, or doula can help you learn these basics before you have to do them by yourself. It will take a little practice to feel you know what to do. Your baby will be okay while you learn. The most important thing is to be gentle and loving with your baby.

Feeding your newborn

Your baby knows how to suck. She has been sucking her fingers in the uterus. Offer her your breast right after birth. She may want to latch on right away. But, it is also normal if baby doesn't want to breastfeed very much at first.

The nurses or a breastfeeding expert (lactation consultant) can help you get started. If you have questions, be sure to ask before you go home.

To get breastfeeding off to a good start:

◆ Hold your baby so her tummy is against yours.

◆ Touch her top lip with your nipple.

◆ Make sure her mouth is wide open and her lips out. The nipple and most of the dark areola will fit inside.

◆ Let her nurse often. Her stomach is too small to hold much milk at once.

◆ Ask the nurses not to give her water or formula. That will make her less hungry for breast milk.

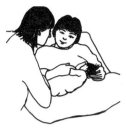

A lactation consultant can help you with breastfeeding.

If you bottle feed, give only very small amounts at first. Newborns have very small stomachs. Eating too much can cause problems.

For a whole chapter on feeding, read Chapter 12.

Ways to hold and comfort baby

◆ **Cuddling:** Babies love to be held. Cuddle your baby against your chest so she can hear your heart beat, feel your warmth, and smell your body. Gently pat or rub her back.

◆ **Kangaroo care:** Your new baby may like being held with her skin against your bare chest. Put a light blanket over both of you. This is called kangaroo care. It is especially good for preemies and can help them develop well. This closeness also helps get your milk supply started.

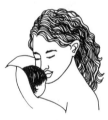

Skin-to-skin time (kangaroo care) is very good for young babies.

◆ **Moving:** Babies love to be rocked and walked. It gives them the same feeling they had in your uterus. Remember to keep one hand behind baby's head. Her neck isn't strong enough to hold up her heavy head.

◆ **Sounds:** Babies like high, sing-song sounds. They like the beat of songs. Talk to your baby in a soft voice. This kind of baby talk is natural and helps them learn. You can use real words or gentle sounds.

◆ **Sucking:** This is comforting to a baby even when she is not hungry. Wash your hands and let her suck on your little finger.

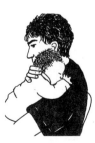

Keep your hand behind baby's head when holding her.

For many details on how babies behave, read Chapter 13.

First steps of baby care

Keeping her warm

New babies are used to the warmth of your body. Keep your baby's body covered lightly indoors. Swaddling keeps her cozy.

She will need a sweater or blanket only if the room is cool. She could get too hot if covered with too many blankets. When you go outside in cold weather, add a hat and a blanket or snowsuit.

How can you tell if your baby is warm enough? Her back and tummy should feel warm like your body but not hot or sweaty. It is normal for a baby's face, hands and feet to feel cool.

Swaddling

Your baby may like being wrapped snugly in a thin blanket. (See pictures below.) Swaddling helps her feel secure, the way she was in your belly. Wrap her snugly around her body but keep the blanket loose around her legs. She needs to be able to bend her knees. You can leave her hands out so she can suck on her fist. (You also could buy a swaddle sack.)

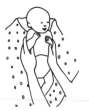 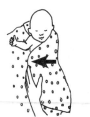 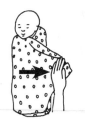

1. Place baby's head at one corner of a receiving blanket.

2. Bend her knees, then wrap one corner around and tuck it in.

3. Pull the bottom corner up to her chest.

4. Finally, wrap the other corner over her arms.

5. Tuck corner of blanket under your baby.

Swaddling your baby with feet loose

Keeping her clean

Change your baby's diaper often to protect her tender skin. Some babies cry when they are being changed. They may feel cold when they are naked.

It is good to check baby's diaper often. Wet diapers tell you she is getting enough breast milk or formula. After feeding is going well, she should have at least 6 to 8 wet diapers each day.

Your newborn's first few bowel movements (stool or poop) are thick and black. This is called meconium and it is normal. The next few stools will be greenish. After that, they will be yellow. She probably will have 3 to 4 dirty diapers a day at first.

Be sure to wash your hands well with soap before and after changing her diaper.

Keeping germs away

Wash your hands often when caring for your baby. Make sure that others who care or play with her also wash their hands first. Even if hands look clean, they can carry germs.

Keep your new baby away from people with colds or other illnesses she might catch. It's best not to take your baby into crowds, such as stores or parties, until she is older. This is especially important if she is a preemie or has any breathing problems.

Keeping her safe

The most important safety concerns with new babies are injury in car crashes and during sleep. Sleep problems are Sudden Infant Death Syndrome (SIDS) and suffocation*.

*Suffocation: Breathing blocked by pillow, quilt, cushions, or position against a wall.

Sleep safety basics:

- Always put your baby to sleep on her back unless there is a medical reason not to.
- Have her sleep in the same room with you but in her own safe bed (crib or bassinet).
- Use a firm mattress and keep pillows, quilts, and toys out of the crib.

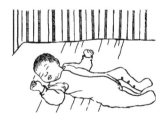

- Dress her warmly and keep the room comfortably cool. She should be warm but not hot.
- Keep her away from smoky places.
- Breastfeed her.

Car safety basics:

- Make sure to use a car seat on every car ride.
- Install the car seat tightly in the back seat, facing the back of the car.

◆ Buckle the harness over both shoulders and between her legs.

◆ Make straps snug.

For many important details about safety, read Chapter 14.

Know the signs of health problems

Read Chapter 15, pages 236–237, for signs of serious illness that you need to know. These things probably won't happen. But if they do, you must be ready to take your baby to her provider.

Do not wait for any of these problems to get better by themselves. Call right away.

Circumcision

If your baby is a boy, you will need to decide if you want him circumcised or not. If you want it, it is done soon after birth, so it's good to decide before baby comes.

What is circumcision surgery like?

Uncircumcized (intact) penis

At birth, the skin on the penis covers all the way over the tip. Circumcision is a minor surgery that cuts part of the skin off to uncover the tip of the penis. It does hurt, but they can use drugs to help.

After surgery, you must take care of the cut while it heals. This usually takes about a week. There are small chances of infection or other problems.

Why or why not to circumcise?

Circumcized penis

Some parents choose to circumcise due to religious beliefs or because they value the health benefits later on. Others choose not to circumcise because they don't want their baby to have painful surgery. Many want their son's penis to look like his dad's or look the same as other boys in school.

Circumcision is not usually covered by health insurance. Check before you decide.

There are health benefits of circumcising, but they are not great. Talk to your provider and ask questions. You may also want to find out if it's covered by your insurance. Decide what feels right to you and your partner.

Going home

If both you and your baby are doing well, you will probably be able to go home within a day or two after delivery. Being at home will give you more rest and keep you away from germs.

Before You Take Your Baby Home

- ☐ Know whom to call if you or your baby has a health problem.
- ☐ Get the name and phone number of a breastfeeding expert (lactation consultant).
- ☐ Make sure your baby has started to breastfeed well. Know how to get her to suck on the nipple (latch on) properly. Practice squeezing (expressing) a small amount of milk out of your nipples with your fingers.
- ☐ Buckle your baby's car seat into the back seat for the ride home. Take off swaddling blankets before putting baby in the car seat.
- ☐ Make an appointment to bring your baby for her first checkup. This is usually between 1 and 3 days after going home.

If you have had a c-section, you will need to stay longer to recover. If your baby is very small or had problems at birth, she will probably have to stay longer, too.

Making the first ride a safe ride

One of the most important things is to buckle up your baby right in his car seat. If you have a small seat with a handle, you can buckle up baby inside your room. Then carry baby in it to the car. If the seat has a base or is a convertible, install that in the car first.

Take off any swaddling blankets. Make sure the harness goes over both shoulders and between her legs. The shoulder straps should be at or below baby's shoulders, if possible. Make the straps snug. If the weather is cold, wrap a blanket over her after the harness has been adjusted. See Chapter 14 for more about car seat safety.

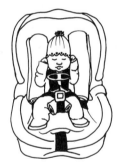

Baby ready to go home in her car seat.

If you go home by taxi, be sure the driver gives you time to get the car seat properly installed, following the instructions.

Support from your health care providers

You can get support by phone or email from your providers and others, day or night. No question is too small to ask.

Make sure to have the phone numbers for support people who you can call.

- ◆ your doctor or midwife
- ◆ baby's doctor or nurse practitioner

◆ lactation consultant

◆ your social worker, local family center, or new mom support group

You may have hired a doula who will visit you and help out for the first few days or weeks. Some lactation consultants and nurses also make home visits. A home visit can be very helpful. Find out if your hospital or health department offers this service.

The first weeks at home

Your first days at home as a family are a very special time. It can also be a hard time. You will be tired and may feel unsure about what to do. The most important thing is to keep giving gentle, loving care to your baby and yourself.

It is also important to get as much rest as possible, so your body can heal. Try to sleep when baby does. Ask others to help you by doing laundry, cooking, grocery shopping, or cleaning. Let them do things for you and your partner so that you can pay attention to your baby.

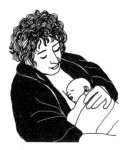

Take the time to relax with baby. Kangaroo care is one of the best ways to help her feel at home in the world.

Holding and carrying your baby

Pick her up as often as she wants. You can't spoil her at this age by holding her too much. Hold your baby skin to skin or against your shoulder, cradle her in one arm, or tuck her feet under your arm (football hold).

When your baby cries, try to figure out what she is telling you. Is she hungry, wet, tired, or lonely? You will learn how to know what she needs. She may just want to be cuddled.

Wearing your baby

One way to have your baby close while you do other things is to put her in a cloth baby carrier. This makes it easy to take a walk, do light housework, or go shopping with your baby. This can be very soothing for a fussy baby or one who doesn't go to sleep easily.

There are many kinds of carriers. You might have to try different kinds until you find one that works well for you. Check how big your baby must be before using it.

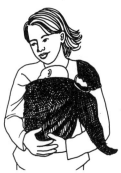

Wearing your baby.

Some carriers are not safe for newborns. Some require an added piece for small babies. Most carriers are not safe for small preemies, so be sure to ask baby's nurse before using one. Find one that fits your body, fits your baby, and is easy to get off and on. Find important safety tips in Chapter 14.

Changing diapers

Baby's bowel movements (poops or stool)

What goes in, must come out. All parents have to clean their baby's bottom, even though it's not much fun.

After your newborn's first stool, they will be yellow. What your baby eats will make stools look different.

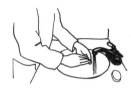

Don't forget to wash your hands after changing baby's diaper.

+ Breast milk makes a light yellow, very soft stool, like lumpy mustard. In the early weeks, a baby may have as many as 10 small stools each day. After 6 weeks she may have one every day or two.

+ Formula makes a tan or yellow stool (about as hard as peanut butter). Baby should have one or two each day.

If the stools are hard and dry, your baby may not be getting enough milk or formula. Call your baby's provider.

Cleaning your baby's genitals*

Always wipe your baby's bottom from front to back. This keeps germs in the stool from getting into baby's penis or vagina. For boys, wipe the penis from base to tip. For girls, gently open the folds of skin around the vagina. Wipe them from front to back.

*Genitals:
A boy's penis or a girl's vulva.

If your baby boy is not circumcised, the foreskin will be tight all the way to the tip. Don't try to pull it back when washing it. It will loosen itself by age 5.

A newborn girl may have some bloody or milky liquid coming from her vagina. This is normal in the first week.

Baby wipes are handy but you don't need to buy them. You can use warm water with cotton balls or small soft washcloths instead. Be sure to clean the washclothes well. It is best not to use baby oil or powder. Although they are sold for babies, they can hurt tender skin. Talcum powder can be very bad for a baby's lungs.

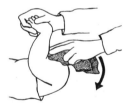

Always clean genitals from front to back.

$$ Use warm water and cotton balls or small washcloths instead of baby wipes.

Care for a boy's circumcised penis

A baby boy's circumcision can take one to two weeks to heal. Fasten diapers loosely. Do not lay your baby on his tummy until his penis has healed. Ask your baby's provider before you put medicine or a bandage on it.

To keep the area clean, wash it very gently when changing diapers. Drip warm soapy water over it. Rinse it with warm clean water and then pat it dry.

Call the doctor or nurse if you see bleeding or signs of infection. Infection causes white pus, redness, and swelling. Also call if your baby has a hard time urinating.

Cord care in the first few weeks

Keep the cord stump clean and dry. Fold the front of each clean diaper down below the stump. Clean the the area around the stump with warm water once a day and if it gets stool on it. Do not put baby's belly under water until a few days after the stump falls off. The stump will get dry and black. Then it will fall off in about a month. It will leave a nice belly button.

Never try to pull the stump off. Call your baby's provider if the skin around it gets red, warm and smelly, or oozes pus.

Diaper rash

*Diaper rash: A painful, red, bumpy rash around the genitals and bottom.

It is easy to prevent diaper rash*.

- ◆ Change your baby's diaper every two or three hours and as soon as possible after each bowel movement.

- ◆ Dry the area well before putting on another diaper.

- ◆ Let your baby lie without a diaper on for a while every day. Lay her naked on her tummy on a waterproof pad covered with a diaper or towel. Make sure the room is warm or put a shirt and socks on her.

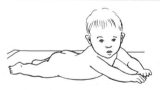

Fresh air helps prevent and calm diaper rash.

If your baby gets a rash, be sure to change diapers more often. Wash the area gently with warm water and pat it dry. Let your baby lie with her bottom bare. Spread a thick baby ointment (such as A & D ointment or zinc oxide cream) on the rash when you change diapers. If it is not better in two or three days, it might be infected. Call her provider.

Bathing your new baby

Use a small wash cloth to clean your baby's face, neck, belly button, and bottom each day. You need to wash her whole body only every few days. As she gets older, you both may enjoy bath time every day.

At first, give a sponge bath. Wait until after the cord has fallen off before putting baby in a tub of water. Also wait until a circumcision has healed.

Babies should always be washed from the top down. Start with the face and hair and end with the bottom. This keeps germs from the bottom away from the face and hands.

Getting ready for the bath

Make sure the room is warm. The kitchen can be a good place for a bath, because you can stand up at the counter.

Collect all the things you need before you start the bath. This is easier than looking for things while your baby is wet and soapy.

Have these things where you can reach them:

- Warm water in bowls or tub. Test it with your elbow or the back of your hand to make sure it is skin temperature.
- Washcloth (and a cup for scooping water in a tub)
- Mild soap or baby wash
- A few towels
- Clean clothes and fresh diaper

Giving a sponge bath

Give a sponge bath on a wide flat counter or table. Have a wash cloth (not a sponge) and two bowls of warm water within reach. One bowl is for washing, so put a bit of soap in it. The other bowl is to rinse your washcloth between body parts. Start with baby wrapped in a towel, unless the room is quite warm.

Washing baby's hair.

- Lay your baby on a clean towel.
- Always keep one hand on her so she will not fall.
- Wash and dry her face and hair first. You can keep her shirt and diaper on when you do this.
- Then start washing her neck and finish with her legs and bottom.
- Wash, rinse, and dry one part of her body at a time. Keep the rest of her body covered to keep her warm.

A tub bath for a slippery baby

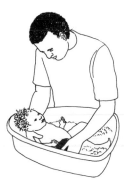

Use a baby tub or put a foam pad or a soft towel in the bottom of the clean kitchen sink. Put a few inches of slightly warm water in the tub. Put a folded towel or foam pad in the bottom to help keep baby from slipping around.

◆ Hold your baby with one arm under her head and shoulders. Hold her arm in that hand.

◆ Wash and rinse with the other hand.

◆ Never leave your baby alone in the bath—even for a second! A baby can drown quickly and silently if left alone.

Baby's skin

A new baby's skin may get very dry. This is normal and usually okay left alone. If you are worried that baby's skin is too dry, you can rub on a mild, unscented skin cream.

"My baby loved to be massaged with oil. It was a little game we played after a bath. I'd tell her how cute her tummy, fingers, and toes were."

Rashes are common in babies, and are usually normal. You can try using soaps that are not scented for baby's skin and laundry.

Some babies have tiny pimples on their face and body. This is also normal and will go away. Don't try to scrub or pop them, and don't use any special soaps or creams.

You may see small brown or yellow flakes under baby's hair. This is called "cradle cap" and is very common. Wash baby's hair normally. You may also use a soft brush and some oil, but don't scrub or pick the scales off. They won't hurt baby and will go away. Ask her doctor or nurse if you are worried.

If your baby has any rash, bumps, or dry spots that seem to be itchy or painful, call her doctor or nurse. Call if you see anything that turns bright red, bleeds, or oozes yellow pus.

Cleaning gums and teeth

Most babies do not get their first teeth until at least four months. Before teeth start coming in, it is good to wipe your baby's gums with a small soft cloth every day. This helps her get used to the feeling of having her mouth cleaned.

When her first teeth start coming in, wipe them daily or use a soft baby tooth brush. If you use any toothpaste, use only a tiny smear (like a grain of rice) on the brush. Ask your baby's doctor or nurse if you should use toothpaste with fluoride once your baby has her first tooth.

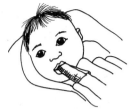

It is important to keep baby teeth healthy. Your baby needs those teeth for many things besides chewing food. Teeth help baby talk. They also hold space in the gums for the adult set of teeth.

"My baby didn't like having his teeth brushed. I wish I had started wiping his gums earlier."

Dressing for inside and outside

Unless your baby is a preemie or very small, your baby needs to wear only a little warmer clothing than you do. Dress her in one layer more than you wear. If your baby is a preemie, she will need another layer unless the room is very warm.

When going outside, put a hat on her. This will help keep her from losing heat through her head. If the weather is very cold or hot, avoid taking her out for the first few weeks.

Heavy blankets can make your baby too hot inside. Unless your baby is very small (less than about 4½ pounds) or is out in cold weather, she does not need to be covered with thick blankets. Thin blankets are also safer for baby's breathing.

Protect your baby from the sun

Try to keep your baby out of direct sun for the first six months. It's very easy for her to get sunburned, whether her skin is light or dark. Keep your baby in the shade when you can, especially between 10 a.m and 4 p.m. The sun can burn even on cloudy days. Sun is especially bright at the beach or where there is snow on the ground.

If baby's provider says that sunshine may help her jaundice, ask how to do it safely.

If there is no shade, dress your baby in light colored clothes that cover her up. A sun hat with a wide brim will also help protect her. Use a sunscreen made for babies rated SPF 15 or more. Put it on any skin that is showing. Don't forget the face, ears, and the back of her hands. Put more on often.

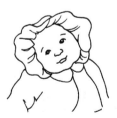

A sun hat with a brim.

If your baby needs special health care

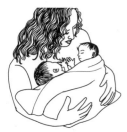

Even if baby is in an isolette, you can help by touching and talking softly to her.

Some newborn babies are born with a birth defect or a problem like low birth weight or being premature. Some problems are more serious than others.

You may never know why the problem happened. Try not to blame yourself. Instead, focus on helping baby get well.

If your new baby needs to stay in the hospital, she is likely to be kept in the newborn intensive care unit. There she can get the special care she needs. It will have dim lights, be warm, and be as quiet as possible. These things help a baby keep growing and developing well. (Twins or multiples may be kept together.)

While your baby is in the NICU, spend a lot of time with her if possible. She needs to hear your voice and feel your touch. This is as important as all the tubes, machines, and medicines. Try to help with her care as much as her health allows. This is a good way for you and your partner to learn how to care for her when she comes home.

Learn about her condition

Find out when "rounds" are on your unit. This is when your baby's doctors will come by each day.

- ◆ Try to be at the NICU when the doctor checks your baby. This is the best time to ask about what's happening. You also can learn a lot from the NICU nurses.

  - ▶ Find out as much as possible about the condition your baby has. Ask the hospital social worker for help getting information. See Chapter 17 for resources.

  - ▶ If you are not sure a specific treatment is best for your baby, ask for a second opinion. It is always OK to ask for another doctor's advice.

Comforting your baby

Kangaroo care, holding baby skin to skin against your chest, can be very healing for your baby. It helps her feel connected to you, breathe well, and stay calm. It also helps you bond with baby. Your partner and other family members can also do kangaroo care if her doctors allow.

Kangaroo care for tiny twins.

Many babies can be breastfed in the NICU. But you may have to wait a few days or weeks before baby is able to nurse. Start pumping right away so your breasts will make milk. In many cases, that milk can be given to baby in a bottle until she can nurse. Skin-to-skin time may help your milk come in during this time. Ask for a breastfeeding consultant to help you.

Dealing with your feelings

If your child has a health problem at birth, it often is a big surprise. Parents whose baby is not born exactly the way they expected often feel very scared, sad, guilty, or angry. These feelings are normal. Here are some ways you can cope:

"When my baby was tiny, both her father and I loved holding her against our bare chests. She really seemed happy there."

- Spend as much time as possible with your baby.

- Talk with the social worker about your feelings. The social worker can tell you about parent support groups. Partners may also want support to get through this difficult time.

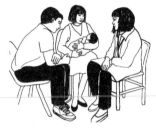

Modern medical care helps many babies with special needs to lead healthy, happy lives. Your baby will need your love and attention, just like any other baby. Caring for her can be very hard and also very rewarding.

See Chapter 15 for details on caring for a sick baby.

Tips for partners

- **Touch your baby.** Hold her, talk to her, let her sleep on your bare chest. This is good for her and will help you get to know each other.

- **Support your partner.** She may be very emotional, with good feelings or with worries. Be kind and loving.

- **Help care for baby.** Change diapers, swaddle her, or get her dressed. Be the master of burping or giving baths. Rock or walk with your baby while mom rests.

- **Talk to baby's provider.** You can help by asking questions. You can make notes of what the doctor, nurse, or midwife says. Help by keeping track of paperwork and phone numbers.

- **Let people help.** These first weeks are hard. Tell people what they can do. Let them bring you meals, walk the dog, or mow the lawn. Let them help you, so you can help mom and baby.

- **Take pictures now.** The first months go by so quickly. Your baby will change before your eyes. Make sure you have photos to remember this special time.

Chapter 12

Feeding Your New Baby

Your most important job

Feeding time is special. It is not just about filling baby's tummy. It's also about baby feeling close to someone in this big, strange world. When a parent responds quickly to baby's needs, the baby starts to learn to trust people. If a parent makes baby wait, he learns that people may not help him.

A baby will be happiest and grow best if he is fed as soon as he show signs of hunger. Your baby needs more food some days than others. Feed him when he starts to act hungry. When he is growing fast, he will get hungry more often. Watch for his signs of hunger.

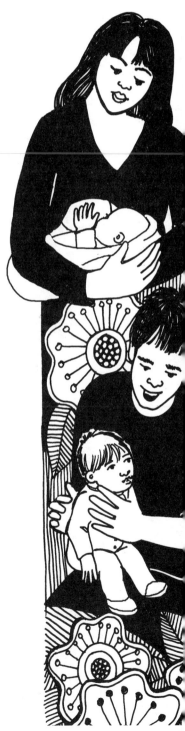

Look in this chapter for:

Basics of feeding from breast or bottle, page 182

Breastfeeding: Getting started, page 184

    Learning to breastfeed

    Eating right while you are nursing

    Ways to hold your baby, nursing twins

    Get help for problems right away

Going back to work or school, page 192

Feeding with a bottle, page 193

    Using baby formula

Tips for partners, page 196

Basics of feeding from breast or bottle
Follow the hunger signs

Try to feed your baby before he starts to cry. Crying isn't the first sign that he's hungry. Watch for these signs:

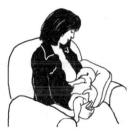

- ◆ Smacking his lips or sticking out his tongue
- ◆ Sucking on his hand
- ◆ Making little soft sounds
- ◆ Turning his head toward your breast when you hold him

It's important for a new baby to feed every two or three hours. Some newborns are very sleepy and need to be waked up to feed. You can wake him gently by talking to him, changing his diaper, taking off some of his clothes, rubbing his back, or sitting him up.

Making feeding a special time

"The quieter the room, the better he eats. Now I turn off the TV and put my phone on silent. It's a lot easier to relax and he's happy."

Feeding can take some time, so make sure you both are comfortable before you begin. Place a firm pillow in your lap to support your arm and your baby. Have a glass of water and a snack next to you. If you want to listen to music, make it very calm and quiet.

Pay attention to your baby while you are feeding him. Look in his eyes and smile. Talk softly or sing a song. Take this time to help him feel safe and loved.

How do you know when he is full?

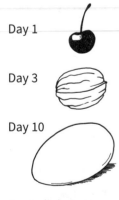

Day 1

Day 3

Day 10

A new baby's stomach is very small but grows fast.

Babies usually know when they are full. Your baby's tummy is very small, as these pictures show. He won't be able to eat very much at a time. That's why he needs to eat so often.

Stop when your baby acts full. Giving your baby too much food will upset his tummy and be frustrating for both of you.

Some signs that he has had enough:

- ◆ He stops sucking and doesn't need to burp.
- ◆ He turns his head away from the breast or the bottle.
- ◆ He starts to fall asleep.

If your baby gets sleepy after only a few minutes of feeding, you can try to help him wake up. Sit him up, burp him, or change his diaper. Then offer him the nipple again. But if he doesn't want it, wait a while.

If you are bottle-feeding, don't try to get your baby to finish a bottle. Let him tell you how much he needs.

For details about bottle-feeding, see page 193.

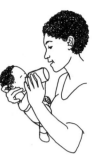

Is baby getting enough to eat?

Feed your baby as much as he wants when he is hungry. Here are some signs that he is getting enough:

- He has at least six wet diapers and at least 3 poopy diapers every 24 hours. His poop should be soft.

- He is gaining weight after the first week.

- He is tired or peaceful after eating and burping.

A baby under 4 to 6 months of age should get enough nutrition from breast milk or formula. He should not need any other food. In fact, even water can be dangerous for babies under 6 months.

Baby can be with you at meal time. When he sits up on his own and seems to want your food, he may be ready to try some of his own. Talk to his provider about when to start foods.

"My mom told me he would sleep better if I put rice cereal in his bottle at night. His doctor said that's not good for him, though."

Burping is part of feeding

Babies often swallow air while eating. You may need to burp him in the middle of a feeding and at the end.

There are lots of ways to burp a baby. You can hold your baby up by your shoulder or on your chest. You can sit him up or lay him on his tummy in your lap. Pat or rub his back gently for a few minutes. Use a cloth to protect your clothes in case he spits up some milk with the burp.

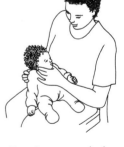

Warning: If your baby vomits forcefully, so liquid shoots several feet out of his mouth, he might have a serious problem. Call the doctor or nurse right away.

Burping a new baby. Sit him on your lap or lay him on your shoulder. Rub or pat his back.

Breastfeeding: Getting Started

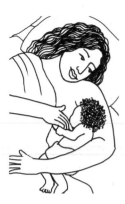

Breast milk is specially made for babies' needs. The milk your breasts make during the first few days is especially nutritious. Breast milk changes as your baby's needs change. (For more about why breastfeeding is important, see Chapter 6.)

A baby does not need other foods for at least 6 months. Wait until he shows interest in foods you are eating. Make sure he can sit up and swallow well before offering other foods. The Academy of Pediatrics advises feeding only breast milk for at least 6 months.

Most babies are ready to nurse right after birth. Many moms love nursing their babies during the first hour or two. But, drugs given to some moms during labor can make their baby sleepy or not hungry right away. If this happens, don't worry. Your baby will be ready soon.

Help learning to breastfeed

Are you taking any medications or supplements? Check with your provider to make sure they don't get into your breast milk and pass to baby.

Breastfeeding is something that you and your baby learn to do together. The most important things are to have baby in a good position that he gets your nipple into his mouth right. If you and your baby have trouble getting started, be sure to ask for help. As you both get used to nursing, it will be much easier.

Be sure to get help right away if you have any concerns. Most new moms who have early breastfeeding problems can get over them and nurse happily.

Who can help you? In the first few days, the nurses or your midwife will be there to help you. Also ask your doctor or midwife for the name and phone number of a lactation (breastfeeding) consultant. Then you will know who to call if you have any questions later on.

Lactation consultants have special training and experience with helping nursing moms. Lactation consultants who are certified have "IBCLC" after their names.

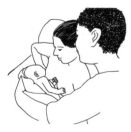

A lactation consultant can give you hands-on help.

You also can call a local member of a breastfeeding group, such as La Leche League (see Chapter 17). Leaders and members are women who have nursed their babies. They can give you their wisdom and support.

You may hear some moms say that they stopped nursing because they didn't have enough milk or baby didn't like it. But usually they didn't get support from a lactation consultant to solve their problems. Today, U.S. health insurance is required to pay for lactation consultants.

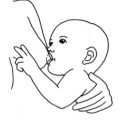

Your breasts are like milk factories

Your breasts will be larger when they are making milk regularly. Your nipple and areola may also be larger and darker. Even if your breasts aren't big, they still make breast milk.

Inside your breasts are the glands that make milk. They will feel like lumps all around your breast area. You may even feel them by your armpits. Tubes (ducts) carry the milk from the glands to your nipples.

"I love how my baby strokes my breast with his hand. He looks like he's dreaming."

After your baby starts sucking, you may feel your breasts "let down." That is when the milk starts to flow from the glands. After a few minutes, the milk gets richer. It is important to let your baby suck on each breast as long as he's still drinking and swallowing. This means he will get the best milk. (This also is important when pumping your breasts.)

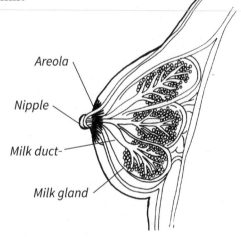

Areola

Nipple

Milk duct-

Milk gland

When your milk "comes in"

During pregnancy, your breasts will start to make colostrum*. It is thick and clear or yellowish. This milk is loaded with antibodies to protect baby from illness.

*Colostrum: The first milk from the breasts.

Two or three days after birth, your breasts will begin to fill with regular breast milk. It is white or bluish-white. It also has lots of antibodies. You will feel your breasts get full. This is normal and can last for a few days.

If they feel too full (engorged), let baby nurse more often. This will keep your breasts from getting too full. Put warm cloths on your breasts or massage them before nursing. This helps the milk flow.

If the areola gets too hard to fit into baby's mouth, you can squeeze (express) a little milk out. This will make it easier for him to fit the nipple in his mouth.

Expressing milk

Expressing breast
milk by hand.

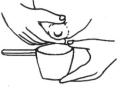

To express milk, press on your breast gently but firmly with your fingers. (See pictures, left.)

1. Massage from all sides toward the areola.

2. Then hold your thumb above and fingers below the areola.

3. Squeeze and release it a few times. A little milk will come out.

Once the areola is soft, baby will be able to latch on. Nursing every few hours helps keep your breasts from getting engorged.

Your breasts will feel best when your baby sucks well and empties them often. After you have been breastfeeding for a few days, they will get softer and feel more comfortable between feedings. They are getting used to making milk.

Eating right while you are nursing

Breast milk is the most nutritious milk for your child. It will be even better if you drink water and eat plenty of:

◆ Calcium from milk, leafy vegetables, and dried beans

◆ Vitamin D, from sunlight and foods with added D

◆ Protein from low-fat meats, eggs, fish, dried beans, nuts

◆ Iron from meat, fish, leafy vegetables, fortified cereals

◆ Folic acid from leafy vegetables, beans, oranges, meat, and folic acid pills.

How often should baby feed?

Is a disposable diaper wet? It can be hard to know. You can tell by holding it up to the light and comparing it to a dry one. Or put a piece of tissue in the diaper. The tissue will feel wet.

◆ After the first day, a baby under 2 months old needs to nurse every one to three hours. This is at least eight to twelve times in 24 hours. Some may eat more often during one part of the day than another.

◆ If your new baby sleeps for more than four hours, it is important to wake him up gently to eat.

To know your baby is getting enough to eat, make sure he is nursing often and well and seems to be happy after nursing. He should wet his diaper at least 6 times each day. Check it often if you are concerned.

Ways to hold your baby for breastfeeding

Get comfortable. You might need to stay this way for a long time. It's good to use different positions for different feedings.

In all these positions, use pillows to make yourself and your baby comfortable. Remember to put baby's tummy flat against your body.

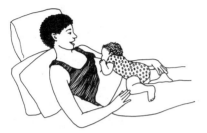

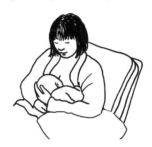

Laid-back hold: *Rest against pillows. Put baby on his tummy with his head on top of your breast and his body on your tummy.*

Football hold: *Sit in a chair and hold your baby next to your side, with legs under your arm. Baby doesn't lie on your tummy. This is a comfortable way to nurse if you have had a c-section.*

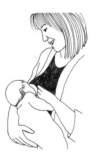

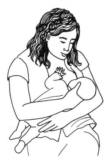

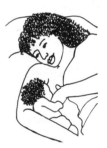

Cradle hold: *Sit in an armchair. Hold your baby across your chest. His head should be in the bend of your arm. Put a firm pillow under your baby's body and your arm.*

Cross-cradle hold: *Sit in an armchair. Hold your baby across your chest. One hand should be at baby's head with your elbow by his bottom. Put a firm pillow under your baby's body and your arm.*

Side-lying hold: *Lie in bed on your side. Lay baby on his side next to you, in the bend of your elbow or on the bed.*

Is your baby getting enough breast milk?

Your breasts almost always can make enough milk for your baby's needs. When baby is hungry, he will suck more and they will make more milk. They can make enough to feed twins!

Every few weeks your baby will probably have a growth spurt*. When this happens, he will want to nurse more often for a couple of days. That will build up your milk supply.

*Growth spurt: A time when baby grows faster than usual. He will suck more to get more nutrition.

Basics of Happy Breastfeeding

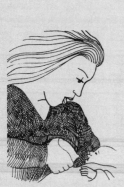

Breastfeeding is natural. Once you get started, it usually is a very happy experience. Follow these basic steps:

◆ Hold your baby so his tummy faces your body. Think "tummy to tummy." His head should face your nipple, so he doesn't have to turn his head to reach it.

◆ Support your breast outside the areola with your thumb on top.

Hold your breast and pull him to it when he opens his mouth.

◆ Get your baby to open his mouth wide by touching his lip with your nipple. Open your mouth—he may do it too.

◆ When he opens his mouth wide, pull him toward you. Guide the nipple and areola deeply into his mouth.

◆ Make sure he gets part of the areola into his mouth. Sucking only on the nipple will not work. Make sure his lower lip is out and the tip of his nose touches your breast. He still will be able to breathe.

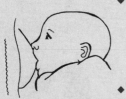

◆ Make sure he is swallowing. He will not swallow every time he sucks. You may hear him gulp or see the skin in front of his ears move a little.

Baby's lower lip should be turned out.

◆ Let baby decide how long to nurse on the first breast. When his sucking slows, burp him and switch breasts. Let him nurse from both breasts at each feeding.

◆ Start the next feeding with the breast he sucked last.

◆ You might need to get the nipple out while he's sucking. Put your finger gently into the corner of his mouth. This breaks the suction without hurting your nipple.

"At first I couldn't remember which breast to begin with. Then I started clipping a little safety pin on my bra strap on the side my baby sucked last. That made life easier."

If your nipples start to get sore, make sure:

◆ Your baby is lying facing your chest

◆ His head is not turned to the side

◆ He has as much nipple and areola in his mouth as possible

◆ Get help! See Chapter 17 for resources.

Using shared breast milk

Feeding your baby another mom's milk can be risky. If you are worried that you aren't making enough milk, talk with your provider or a lactation consultant.

Before using any shared milk, make sure you know:

◆ The health of the person it came from.

◆ How clean the breast milk is.

◆ How fresh it is.

Do you want to share milk? If you are making more milk than you think your baby needs, talk with a lactation consultant. You could give it to a non-profit milk bank for a baby in need.

Wait to give a pacifier or bottle

If your new baby is starting to breastfeed, a pacifier or bottle can hurt, not help. Here's why:

◆ Sucking builds up your supply of breast milk.

◆ A bottle or pacifier nipple could confuse your baby. Those nipples are very different from your breasts. Milk flows out of a bottle much easier. Your baby might start to like the bottle better.

◆ Formula or water can take away his appetite for breast milk.

Most babies love to suck, even when they are not hungry. For now, it's best to offer only your breast or your clean finger. Wait to use a pacifier or a bottle (breastmilk or formula) until he is nursing well. This is often between 4 and 6 weeks of age.

Breastfeeding twins

You can breastfeed your twins. You may want to feed them one at a time at first. As you and the babies get used to nursing, you can feed both at once. This will save you a lot of time. Your breasts will make enough milk for both babies if you nurse often. Give them lots of time to suck.

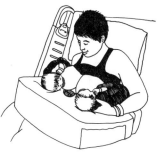

If twins or triplets are born very early, you may need to use special ways to feed them breastmilk. A lactation consultant can help.

Giving vitamins or other supplements?

In most ways, breast milk is the only food your baby needs now. But, breast milk does not contain much vitamin D or fluoride. Ask your baby's doctor or nurse about giving your baby those supplements. After 6 months, your baby may need extra iron. He can get that from solid foods.

Get help for problems right away

If you are having a problem with nursing, ask for help now. Please don't just stop breastfeeding or wait until it gets worse. Call your doctor, midwife, nurse, lactation consultant, WIC nurse, or a La Leche League member for advice. They can give you tips and support to help with most problems.

Some problems that you should call about:

$$ You can use olive oil as a low-cost nipple cream or to massage your breasts and your baby.

◆ Cracked or sore nipples

◆ A hard, red area of your breast that feels warm

◆ A very sleepy baby who does not wake for feedings

◆ Less than 6 wet diapers in 24 hours

If you can't start right away

Sometimes baby can't breastfeed for a few days or weeks because of a medical problem. Usually, a baby get mom's breast milk from spoon, syringe, tube, or a bottle for a few days or even a few weeks. Even if your baby must be given formula for a while, it is often possible for him to learn to nurse later.

If you can't start nursing right after birth, talk to the nurse, lactation consultant, doctor, or midwife as soon as possible. They can help you get set up to pump your breasts until your baby can nurse. Your milk is best—even during the first few days of life. So start pumping right away. If you don't pump, your breasts will stop making milk. Later, it could be very hard to get milk started.

Caring for your breasts

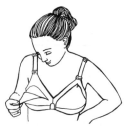

A nursing bra has flaps that open for nursing.

Nursing bras and nursing tank tops can be useful and comforting. If your breasts are heavy, find a bra that is strong enough to support them. If your breasts are naturally small, a nursing tank top may be enough support.

Wash your breasts normally when you bathe. You don't need to wash before or after feeding. Too much soap or washing too often can make your nipples sore.

If your nipples feel sore:

◆ Check to make sure your baby is latching on well. He should lie with his tummy flat against your body.

◆ Vary baby's position for different feedings. That means he will not always suck on your nipples in the same way.

◆ Put a tiny bit of breast milk, lanolin, or nipple cream on your nipples after nursing. This helps healing.

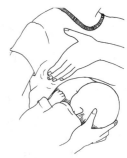

A stretchy bra may be comfortable around the house or at night.

Engorged breasts

If your breasts get very hard (engorged), it can be painful. This can happen if you miss a feeding or stop nursing suddenly. If it lasts for more than a day or you have a fever, talk to your doctor, midwife, or a lactation consultant. Here are some ways to feel better:

◆ Nurse as long as your baby will suck. Let him suck all your milk out.

◆ Squeeze a bit of milk out before your baby latches on.

◆ Use a cool pack for 15 minutes after you nurse. You can put a wet washcloth in the refrigerator to cool.

◆ A warm wet towel might feel good.

One way to help the milk flow through the milk glands in your breasts into the nipple is to massage your breasts gently with your fingertips as your baby sucks. This may help prevent ducts from getting blocked.

A blocked duct will feel like a sore lump in your breast. Massage the area and put a warm washcloth on it before nursing. Those can help the milk flow through it. Let your baby nurse on that breast first. Gently massage the lump while your baby sucks.

Call your provider or a lactation consultant right away if:

◆ A nipple cracks or starts bleeding.

◆ A duct stays blocked for 2 to 3 days.

◆ Your breast has an area that is warm and painful, and you have fever, headache, or flu-like symptoms. These are signs of mastitis*.

Massaging your breasts helps the milk flow.

*Mastitis:
An infection in the breast tissue.

Going back to work or school

Breastfeeding for as long as possible is best for your baby. It also helps your body recover from pregnancy. But remember, any amount of breastfeeding is much better than not doing it at all.

Many women who go back to work outside their home find they can continue breastfeeding. They look forward to the special nursing time when they get home.

To keep up your milk supply, you would use a breast pump at work. Pumping may seem strange at first, but it can give you a lot of milk quickly. The goal is to pump as many times as your baby would nurse if you were with him. Store the milk in a refrigerator or cooler. Take it home for use the next few days or freeze it for later. You can nurse your baby before leaving in the morning and when you are with him again.

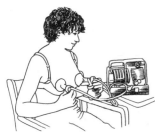

A breast pump looks funny but works well. You can do this in a private place at your job site.

There are pumps that you squeeze with your hand and electric pumps (see picture). Your insurance should cover an electric breast pump. WIC can also provide a pump for moms.

If you work for a company with 50 or more workers, your employer should give you a private place to pump. You should be given breaks to do it during your shift. This is the law, but you may need to talk with your employer to get what you need.

Even if you work in a smaller place, talk with your boss. Ask your boss for a place to pump. Tell him or her that breastfed babies are sick less. That means you won't have to stay home often to care for your sick baby. (See Chapter 12.)

Giving a bottle of breast milk

Many breastfeeding moms want their baby to learn to take a bottle. This allows mom to be away from home for more than an hour or two and to go back to work.

It is best to wait until your baby is nursing well (by about 4 to 6 weeks). Then start offering breast milk in a bottle once a day. Don't wait until just before you go back to work or school. Give baby time to get used to this new way of feeding. Start with a newborn nipple that has a slow flow. That will be most like your breast.

Your baby may learn to take a bottle easier from your partner, a friend, or a grandparent. (He expects you to give him your breast.) If he is not interested in the bottle, try slipping it into his mouth just as he is waking up. He will soon understand that a bottle is just another way to get his favorite food, your milk.

Whenever your baby gets your milk from a bottle, it's best to pump your breasts. This will help your milk supply keep up. If your breasts skip a feeding, they will make less milk.

Feeding with a Bottle

Whether you are using a bottle for breast milk or formula, make feeding time special. Hold your baby against your body with his head higher than his tummy. Look at him and talk softly.

It is very important to hold your baby. Do not prop up the bottle and leave him alone. Your baby needs the feeling of closeness he gets during feeding. He needs this time with you or other caregivers. Also, he could choke if left alone with a bottle. Make sure all baby's caregivers know to hold baby.

Using baby formula

Some moms prefer not to nurse. There may be a medical reason not to. If you feed your baby formula, he can still grow up very healthy. If you are not breastfeeding at all, you will have to stop your breasts from making milk. (See the last page in this chapter.)

Choosing a baby formula

- Always use formula, not plain milk. Formula is made to be as much like breast milk as it can be. Plain cow's milk, soy, rice, or condensed milk do not have all the right nutrients for your baby.
- Most babies do well on a formula based on cow's milk. If you think your baby has a problem with that, talk with his doctor before trying another kind.
- Choose a formula with iron unless your baby's provider tells you not to.

"My three-month-old didn't want to take a bottle. My mom and I decided to try offering a bottle when he was waking up.

She held him while he slept, keeping a bottle of breast milk next to her chair. When he started to wake up, she popped the nipple into his mouth and he began to suck. After that, he took bottles happily when I went to work."

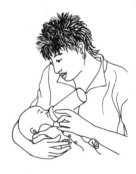

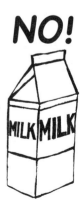

Become a Bottle Expert

Whether you are feeding breast milk or formula, be sure to:

1. Use a fresh bottle for each feeding. Do not keep unused breast milk or formula to finish later. Germs can grow in the bottle, even if you keep it cold.

   Never add water to breast milk. Don't thin formula by adding more water than directions say.

2. Warm the bottle in a bowl of hot water.

   Never heat a bottle in a microwave. The milk (or formula) could get hot and burn your baby's mouth—even if the bottle does not feel hot.

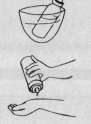

Warming a bottle and testing the temperature of milk

3. Swirl or gently shake the bottle. This makes the liquid all the same temperature.

4. Test the liquid by dripping a little onto the inside of your wrist. It should feel as warm as your skin.

5. Hold baby close, with his head above his body, not flat. Make sure to look at him.

6. Touch your baby's top lip with the nipple so he opens his mouth. Let him take the nipple straight into his mouth. Tip the bottle so milk fills the nipple.

7. Pause after each ounce or two. Burp baby. Stop when he shows you he has had enough.

8. Do not push him to take more than he wants.

9. Wash the bottles and nipples in hot, soapy water after every use. Boil nipples before using for the first time.

Tips about nipples

Newborn nipple with slow flow

+ Nipples come in different shapes. Your baby may like one kind better than others.

+ Make sure the nipple does not flow too fast. Use a newborn nipple with a small hole at first. The milk should come out slowly (see pictures). If your baby starts to cough or choke, the nipple hole is too big.

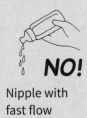

NO!

Nipple with fast flow

◆ Powdered formula is the least expensive but liquid, ready-to-use formula is easier.

◆ If your baby is a preemie or has health issues, powdered formula may not be clean enough. Talk with baby's health care provider about the best kind to use.

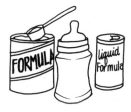

Using formula

◆ To mix powdered formula, follow the directions on the package. Be careful to measure correctly.

◆ Be sure the water is clean. If you aren't sure, use bottled water.

◆ While your baby is a newborn, put only a few ounces in the bottle at one time. Always throw out any formula that he does not drink in one hour.

◆ Do not push your baby to drink more formula than he wants. Generally, a baby under two months of age will want 2 to 4 ounces of formula every 3 to 4 hours.

◆ If you mix the bottles of formula ahead of time, keep them in the refrigerator. Do not let them sit at room temperature. If they are not cold, germs can grow in them.

Be sure not to add too little or too much water to formula. This can be dangerous for baby.

Stopping your breasts from making milk

If you do not breastfeed or pump at all, your breasts will stop making milk. This usually takes about a week and can be painful. Here are some ways to stop breasts from making milk:

◆ Wear a supportive bra, but don't bind (wrap) your breasts tightly.

◆ Put cold (ice) packs on your breasts when they hurt.

◆ Take ibuprofen or other pain relievers as needed, according to the package or your provider.

◆ When your breasts get very full and hard (engorged), you may want to express or pump just enough to make them soft. Use a cold pack afterward.

◆ Some people use cabbage leaves, herbs, or medicine to stop their milk. Ask a lactation consultant, nurse, doctor, or midwife before trying these things.

Tips for partners

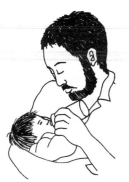

- ◆ Encourage your partner to breast feed as long as possible. It's healthy for baby and costs nothing.

- ◆ Take the lead in bottle feeding when it is time for baby to start learning this new skill. He's likely to take a bottle easier from you than from mom who breastfeeds him.

- ◆ Once baby's taking the bottle, you can do one night feeding so mom can sleep. (Be careful. Dropping a feeding can lower her milk supply. She may need to pump when she wakes up.)

- ◆ Get good at burping baby.

Chapter 13

Getting to Know Your Baby

A newborn baby can do amazing things. Your baby will look at your face. She can hear your voice. She can suck on your breast or your clean finger. She can hold onto your finger.

Think about how new the world is for baby. Until now, she lived curled up in a warm, dark, watery place. She heard the beat of your heart. Now she is in the world of bright lights, sharp noises, cool air, and open space. Loud noises make her jump. Bright lights make her blink. She feels cold when she is undressed. What a lot of change all at once!

Babies start learning about the world as soon as they are born. Their brains grow and learn faster in the first three years than at any other time.

The most important people in your baby's world are you and the others who care for her. Your family will grow together by caring for this new baby.

Look in this chapter for:

A good start for the whole family, page 198
    Partners as parents; moods that get worse
Understanding your new baby, page 200
Talking and playing with baby, page 202
How your baby develops, page 205
    Baby's leaps and delays in learning
Getting baby to sleep, page 207
When baby cries, page 208
    When the crying won't stop
Tips for partners, page 211

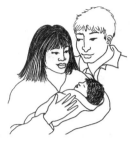

A good start for the whole family

A baby grows best in a happy home. It is important for parents to try to listen to and support each other. Mom will need extra help in the first few months while her body heals and she spends time with the baby. A partner can also need help. Older children will need more attention and love at this time, too.

Your first days as a mom

Your main jobs now are to get to know your baby, feed her, and help your body heal. (For more about your own recovery, see Chapter 15.)

"Feeding time is our special time together. She snuggles in and I sing quietly to her. It helps us both relax."

When you nurse, give your baby plenty of time to feed. Remember, sucking helps build up your milk supply and comforts baby. Nurse her in a quiet place. Have a glass of water and a snack where you can reach them. Use pillows to make sure you and baby are both comfortable.

Take naps or rest when your baby sleeps. Ask your partner, family, and friends to do cooking, shopping, and laundry. If you are tired from too many guests or phone calls, it is okay to say "not now." Ask them to call in a week or two.

You may feel like you don't know how to care for baby. This is a common feeling. You will learn as you go along.

Don't be shy. Ask for help. Nurses, breastfeeding consultants, and others can show you how to do things. But, you don't have to follow all the advice. You are the parent and are learning to know what feels right for you and baby.

Partners as parents

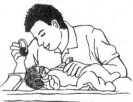

As a partner or husband, you are a key part of the parent team. Mom and baby both need you! You are very important in baby's life. You will learn your own ways of caring for your child.

The more time you spend with your baby, the more comfortable you will feel. Take time to touch, cuddle, and talk to her. She will learn quickly to know your voice, smell, and touch. Hold her close and talk to her quietly in a high, singsong voice. Care for your baby all by yourself sometimes. Soon you will feel comfortable changing her diaper or comforting her.

You and mom will need teamwork to get things done around the house. Use your energy for the most important tasks. Other things like vacuuming or lawn mowing can wait. Take time to rest, eat, and think about all that is going on. It's important to take care of yourself, too.

Watch out for moods that get worse

Feeling tired or having the baby blues is normal in the first few weeks after your baby is born. Many parents get depressed or anxious but it doesn't go away. This can be serious. Watch out for each other. Look for the signs of a mood problem in Chapter 16, page 245.

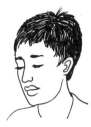

A mood problem can be very serious, but it can also be treated. It's important to get help quickly. If these feelings get in the way of daily life or last more than two weeks, call your provider right away. If your partner isn't able to call herself, call for her.

Older children at home

If you have other children, they may not find your new baby very exciting. The baby will take most of your time. This can make the other kids act needy or angry. This is normal. Here are some ways to help them:

- Spend some special time with each older child every day. Let them know you still love them just as much as before.

- Let older kids "help" you with the baby, but stay with baby at all times. Let your child make funny faces at baby while you change him. Your child isn't old enough to know how to keep baby safe. For example, your 3-year-old may want to carry baby but could drop her by mistake.

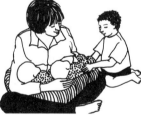

Big brother helping mom.

Don't leave the baby alone with a child under age 12 or 13. Even at that age, some children are not grown up enough to be responsible.

Grandparents and other family members

It is good for babies to get to know their grandparents, aunts, uncles, and cousins. Some family members may help care for your baby a lot.

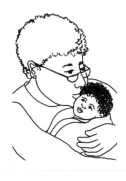

Relatives can be a big help, but they may have outdated ideas of how to care for a baby. They may not believe new baby care advice, like putting baby to sleep on her back or using a car seat. Ask them to learn about and follow the new ways of baby care. If your relatives don't understand, offer this book. It could help them learn new ways to help you.

Remember that you and your partner are the parents. You make the decisions about what is best for your baby. You have tried to learn and use the best information you have found.

If you are a teen, your parents may help care for your baby. You will need to talk to each other a lot about how to care for your baby. There will be many choices to make and it's best if you can all agree. Tell them your reasons for doing things one way. If they don't agree, ask them why. Keep in mind that you all love your baby and want what's best. Your nurse or case worker may be able to help with these talks.

Help with twins, triplets, or more babies

One baby is a lot of work. If you have twins or triplets (or more), you and your partner will need more help. Local groups for new moms about parenting twins can give you very useful advice and support. Look for Mothers of Twins or Multiples groups and other resources listed in Chapter 17.

Understanding your new baby

Your newborn baby can't talk, but she does try to let you know what she wants. Watch what your baby does. You, your partner, and other caregivers will learn what her sounds and expressions mean. This will help you to meet her needs.

How does baby act when sleeping?

- **When she is in a deep sleep,** she breathes slowly and does not wake up easily. This is a good time to move her if you have to, like from car seat to crib.

- **When she is in a light sleep,** her breathing will be less regular. Her eyes may move under their lids. She may move her mouth like she is sucking and move her arms and legs. She may wake easily.

- ◆ **If she starts to wake after sleeping only a short time,** wait a few minutes before picking her up. Put your hand on her chest, whisper "shhh-shhh-shhh," or let her suck on your finger. She may go back to sleep.

How does baby act when awake?

- ◆ **When your baby is waking up** she may need some quiet time before she is ready to eat or play. Talk softly to her, rub her body, and change her diaper.

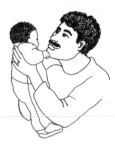

- ◆ **When she is awake and alert** she will look at you and listen to your voice. This is a good time to play.

A newborn baby may only be able to do this for a minute or two at a time. When she looks away or turns her head, that means she needs to rest. Then it's best to just hold her quietly.

- ◆ **If your baby is fussy,** she may need your help to calm down. Make sure you are calm first. Then hold her close and rock her gently or walk her.

- ◆ **When she is hungry,** she may stick her tongue out, suck on her fingers, turn her head toward your body, and make soft sounds. She will be hungry before she starts crying. Try to feed her before she starts crying.

- ◆ **When your baby is getting tired,** her eyes will blink slowly. She will move her arms and legs slowly and make soft noises. She may startle more easily at loud sounds. Try to put her to sleep before she cries.

"When my baby was fussy, I tried playing with her to make her feel better. It only made her cry more. I finally learned that what she needed was quiet cuddling, not more playing."

Every baby's personality is different

Each baby shows signs of his or her own way of behaving from early on. Some are very calm and quiet, watching what is going on around them. Others may be shy. Some are very active and easy to excite. Watch your baby to see what she is like.

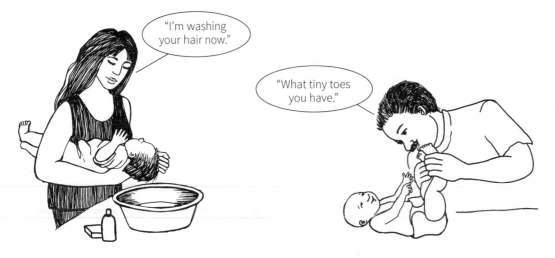

Talking to your new baby

Your baby can hear the sounds around her as soon as she is born. She is getting ready to talk and think long before she knows what words mean.

Hold her close to your face while you talk to her. (See the pictures above.) She will love high sing-song sounds. Talk slowly in a high voice. That helps her hear sounds clearly. You can use real words, not just "baby talk." You can show her a picture book and tell her about the drawings. Or just talk about the things you do all day. Soon she will start making sounds herself ("coo" and later "da-da-da"). When she does this, it is good to make those same sounds back to her. This kind of "talking" back and forth is good for her brain development.

A baby can hear the sounds of all languages in the first six to nine months. If you or any family members speak other languages, it is good for your baby to hear those sounds now.

Playing with your new baby

Playing helps your new baby connect with you and learn. Try these things when she is alert, not tired.

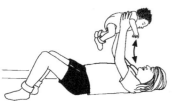

- Hold her 8 to 10 inches from your face. Smile, stick out your tongue, or make a silly face. Watch her face. If she makes a face, do it back at her. It might take a couple of minutes for her to respond. Give her time.
- Lift her gently into the air while looking at her.
- Sing short songs like "Twinkle, Twinkle Little Star."

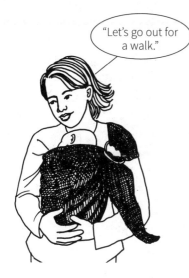

"Let's go out for a walk."

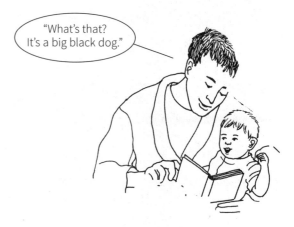

"What's that? It's a big black dog."

- ◆ Touch her gently. Stroke her arms, legs, head, and belly. Rub her feet, hands, and back.
- ◆ Shake a rattle or a bell. Smack your lips, click your tongue, or whistle. See what she does.
- ◆ Show her toys that move or make sounds. Soon she will want to touch and grab them.
- ◆ Hold baby up to look in a mirror.

If your baby was born very early, she may not be ready to play this way until after her due date. Before that time, she just needs to see your face, hear your voice, and feel your arms holding her.

Always play gently—Never, never shake a baby!

Make sure that anyone who plays with your baby always is very gentle. New babies have very large, heavy heads and their necks are weak. Rough play, such as bouncing your baby up and down or tossing her into the air, could hurt her brain seriously.

Tummy time for baby

It is important for every baby, even a newborn, to have some time on her tummy every day. This helps strengthen her neck and arm muscles. She will practice lifting and moving her head. Soon she will start turning it from side to side. Then she will start pushing up with her arms and legs.

Play with your baby on her tummy for a few minutes two or three times a day.

"My baby loved lying on a quilt with big, bright red and yellow ladybugs on it. She would lift her head to look."

- Let her lie on your chest while you lie or sit reclined.
- Lay her on a clean cloth on the floor. A quilt or blanket with a bright pattern will excite her. Turn her head first to one side and then to the other.
- Let her lie on a knit blanket with little lumps in it so she can feel rough textures. She learns a lot by touching.
- Sit or lie down beside her so she can see your face or hands, Talk to her and pat her back. Put small, colorful toys in front of her, so she can try reaching for them.
- Wear her in a carrier when you go out instead of taking her in a stroller.

Sitting up in a play seat, swing, or car seat

The safest way for a new baby to spend time is lying flat on her back or being held. Her neck isn't strong enough to hold her head up. If her head flops forward when sitting up, she might not be able to breathe.

If baby's head flops so her chin is on her chest, wait until she's older before sitting her up. If you do use a play seat or swing, be sure to buckle the safety straps. Keep baby where you can see her.

Make sure her car seat is tilted back enough in the car or stroller so her head doesn't flop.

Take baby out when you get where you're going, even just for a bit. And always keep the straps buckled and snug.

Preventing a flat spot on baby's head

Some babies start to get flat areas on the back of their heads. This can happen if they spend a lot of time lying on their back. This also can come from sitting for long times in a baby seat, car seat, or swing.

If you think your baby might be getting a flat spot, show it to your baby's doctor at the next checkup.

Use the tips below to help her head stay round as she grows. Ways to prevent a flat spot:

- Switch ends of the crib often to help make sure she doesn't always lie with her head on one side.

- Use tummy time for play when she is awake. Put toys on different sides, so she will turn her head.
- Use a baby seat or swing only for short times.
- Use the car seat for travel, not as a place to sleep, eat, or play at home.
- Carry her in a sling or carrier some of the time.

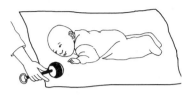

Give baby tummy time every day.

How your baby develops

Watch how your new baby changes. Does she show signs that she can see and hear? Is she learning new things? This is development. Every baby has four kinds of development.

1. Learning to relate to people (like smiling) and trust them (getting comfort from a parent)
2. Physical changes (like rolling over, picking up things with fingers)
3. Thinking and learning (like knowing the faces of people they see often, looking at colors)
4. Language (like letting others know what she wants, making sounds and signs long before she talks)

Baby's development and you

Babies grow best when they feel safe and loved. Every baby's development is closely tied to what parents do, feel, and say. Babies learn trust when parents feed them when they are hungry, and cuddle them when they are upset. This helps baby know that parents will take care of them. It makes them feel safe.

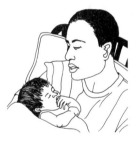

Every new parent needs to learn to respond to their child in a caring way. If you find you have a hard time cuddling, holding, and feeding baby when she needs you, ask for help from your provider.

These early months of baby's life are so important. If you feel depressed, be sure to get help for yourself quickly. Family stress about money or other things can make it hard to give your energy to your baby. Again, tell someone you trust, so you can get help. (See Chapter 16.)

Changes as babies grow and learn

Watch for these signs of change

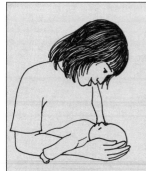

1 week

Most newborns:

- Like to look at a face 8 to 12 inches away
- Follow your face when you move side to side
- React to sounds (by blinking, startling, crying)

At 1 month, most babies:

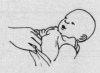

1 month

- Respond to your face and voice
- Turn their head from side to side while on tummy
- Put their hands in their mouths
- Stop crying if picked up and cuddled

At 2–3 months, most babies:

2 months

- Smile when you smile at them
- Turn their head towards sounds
- Make soft cooing sounds
- Lift their head while lying on tummy
- Start to hold up their head when upright
- Calm themselves down some of the time

At 4–5 months, most babies:

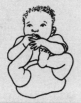

5 months

- Start to roll over from tummy to back
- Smile, laugh, and babble
- Reach for, hold, and put toes in mouth
- Follow a moving toy back and forth with their eyes

At 6–7 months, most babies:

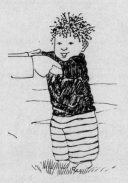

7 months

- Like seeing faces they know, get nervous with strangers
- Smile at themselves in the mirror, know their own name
- Roll both ways, sit up, and stand with support
- Pass toys from one hand to the other

Check out resources in Chapter 17.

Baby's leaps in learning

One of the most exciting things about parenting is watching as baby learns. From week to week you'll see sudden changes. She will have a fussy time for a few days and then suddenly do something new. This is a leap in learning. The first leap usually happens at about 4 to 5 weeks and the next at 8 to 9 weeks. Just before each leap, your baby often needs more attention for a day or two. You may think something is wrong.

After the leap happens, baby will calm down again. You will see her doing some new things at about 5 weeks, like really smiling and looking at things longer. At 9 weeks, she may start playing with her hands and watching people move.

There will be other leaps as baby gets older. Whenever she has a couple of fussy days but isn't sick, watch for her to start doing new things soon.

Watching for delays in development

If you are worried about how well your baby is learning, ask her provider to check. Every baby has her own timetable, but every baby should keep developing. You know your baby best. If you think she is learning too slowly, get help soon. The earlier, the better.

Keep track of baby's changes, new skills, and things that worry you. If you are still concerned, be sure to tell her provider or talk with a nurse or social worker at your public health clinic. Tell them you want baby to have a developmental screening.

A developmental screening is the best way to know how well she's developing. If baby has delays, there are things you can do to help. See Chapter 17 for resources about babies' development.

Getting baby to sleep

Sleep is good for babies. It's also good for parents! But some babies sleep less than others. It can be very hard if yours is one who likes to stay awake.

Getting baby to go to sleep is not always easy. You will hear many ideas about how to do it. There is no one right way for all babies. Try different things to see what works for you and your baby.

> ### Signs that Baby is Ready to Sleep
>
> - She will look away from you, and not want to play.
> - She will yawn, rub her eyes, and make soft, fussy noises.
> - She may have trouble keeping her eyes open.

It may seem easiest to let your baby fall asleep while she is feeding. However, this can become tricky if she gets used to falling asleep in your arms or at your breast. It can be hard to change that habit later.

Do the same things each night to get her ready for bed. Read books, play soft music, and rock her to help her calm down. Start before she seems tired. Try not to wait until she gets really fussy. That usually means she's too tired, making it harder for her to fall asleep.

When you see the sleepy signs, lay her gently on her back in her crib. Make sure her room is quiet and dark. Calm her by rubbing her tummy gently, whispering "shhh . . . shhh . . . shhh." Look away from her or close your eyes. She may fuss a bit, but learning to calm down is part of her development.

If her sleep becomes a problem for you, talk with her provider. And remember, like all things with babies, her sleep will change as the months go on.

When your baby cries

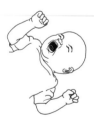

All babies cry. It is normal. It is how they ask for help or tell you that you haven't understood what they wanted. However, crying can make parents feel stressed, worried, or even mad.

Your baby's cry may sound different when she is hungry, tired, wet, lonely, uncomfortable, bored, or sick. You will learn what she is trying to tell you. Even if you don't know the reasons you can try to comfort her. Remember, you won't spoil a baby by picking her up when she cries.

Things that usually calm a crying baby

- Make sure your baby does not have a fever or signs of illness (Chapter 15).

- Change her diaper. Burp her.

- Try feeding her if she hasn't been fed in an hour or more. If she is not hungry, she might like to suck on your clean finger or on a pacifier.

- Swaddle her snugly in a blanket.

- Hold her on her tummy and rock or sway with her.

- Put your baby in a carrier and take a walk inside or outside.

- Try making sounds in her ear, like "shhh, shhh, shhh," over and over again. Some babies like soft singing or dull background noise like the sound of a fan or dryer.

- If she has been awake for a long time, she may be very tired. Try putting her in her crib and patting her tummy lightly or singing. Close your eyes so you don't distract her.

- If your baby cries often and you can't soothe her, talk with her provider to make sure she isn't sick. Some foods may bother her or she may have reflux*.

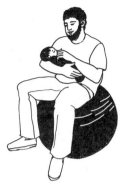

Gentle bouncing can be very soothing for a crying baby.

*Reflux:
Gastroesophageal reflux (GERD), pain that happens if acid from the stomach backs up into the tube from mouth to stomach. There are ways to treat reflux in babies.

When the crying won't stop

In the first few months, some babies have a time most days when they cry hard no matter what you do to calm them. This kind of crying happens most between 2 weeks and 3 to 4 months of age.

If baby doesn't have other signs of being sick, she is likely just fine. Nothing is wrong with her. She just needs to cry a lot. It's normal and it will get better after the first few months. It can be very, very hard for you, though.

What to do? When you know she's not wet, hungry, tired, or sick, here are some other things to try:

- **Music:** Play soft music. Sing or hum along so she hears your voice.

- **Movement:** Dance, sway, rock, or bounce gently.

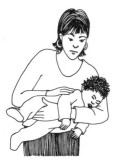

A crying baby may like to be held with your arm under her tummy.

◆ **Cuddle:** Put baby in a carrier so she's held close and facing you. Or, take shirts off and snuggle skin to skin with a blanket wrapped around you both.

◆ **Change things around you:** If you are warm inside, take baby outside where it's cold. If it's quiet, turn on some music. If it's bright, go somewhere dark.

◆ **Get up and go:** Take her for a walk if you need a bit of space. Or, go for a car ride together.

If these things don't work, you haven't failed and baby is okay. You might go back and try all the basics again, like feeding and changing her. If she still doesn't stop crying, you may get very upset. Take a few minutes to take care of yourself.

Get help for yourself when your baby keeps crying

Crying is very hard on the person taking care of baby. When it won't stop, it is very stressful for anyone. You might worry that something is wrong with you or the baby. You might feel like crying, yelling, or shaking.

All of these are signs that you need to take a time out, for your sake and for the baby's. Make a plan for what to do when you have tried everything, baby is still crying, and you are getting upset.

A plan might look like this:

1. Swaddle baby and put her in a safe place like her crib and leave the room. She'll be okay crying in her crib for a few minutes.

2. Take a few deep breaths and put on some music you like to help cover the sound of her crying. Close your eyes.

3. Remind yourself that she isn't choosing to cry. She is not trying to make you mad or hurt you.

"My mom said it's colic, but the doctor said it's not. Nothing's wrong with her body and she doesn't need medicine. She just needs to cry a lot right now. But it's really hard for me."

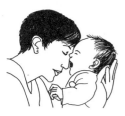

4. Tell yourself you are not doing anything wrong. Call a friend and tell her how frustrated you feel.

5. Put a cool cloth on your face or drink a glass of water. Avoid alcohol or drugs.

6. Remember, this hard time will get better when baby gets a little older.

7. Once you're calm, go back to baby and try again.

You must take care of yourself, too. Ask someone you trust to take care of baby sometimes. Make sure it's someone you know won't get upset if baby cries. Take time to relax or get things done.

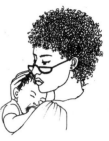

NEVER shake your baby!

It's important to put baby down in a safe place and go into the next room if you feel really upset.

Shaking, hitting, dropping, or throwing a baby can badly hurt her brain. This is called *shaken baby syndrome* or *abusive head trauma*, and it can't be undone. Most of these brain injuries happen when a baby won't stop crying and the adult doesn't put her down in time.

Tips for partners

- Hold your baby. Smile at her and talk to her. Make faces with her. Read a colorful picture book to her. This is how newborns play and learn. She'll be able to play more when she gets a bit older. For now, she will love just watching and being with you.

- Spend time with your partner. You're a family now. It will be important to her that you love and respect her as a mother. It is also good for your baby to see that you care for each other.

- Be patient. This can be a very hard time for you, too. Talk with a friend.

- If your baby cries non-stop for part of the day, remember she'll outgrow it. This is a time when teamwork is most important for you and your partner.

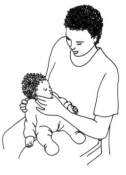

- Take turns caring for baby. You will find your own ways to feed or burp your baby, calm her cries, or get her to sleep. It is good for you and baby to have time together. It's also good for mom to get a break.

- You can have fun giving her a bath. Afterward, massage her legs and arms with olive oil.

- Watch out for signs of mood problems. Be honest and kind with your partner. Speak up if you are worried. These illnesses can happen to partners, too. Talk to someone about your feelings. Ask for help when you need it.

Chapter 14

Keeping Your Baby Safe

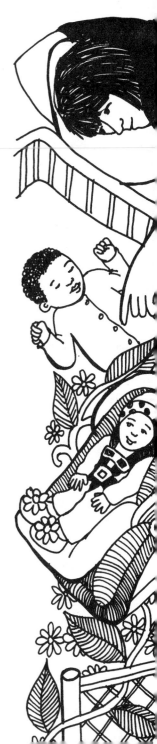

It's scary to think about anything happening to your new baby. Learn how to protect him now. This means you can worry less. For healthy babies, the biggest dangers in the first year are:

- SIDS (Sudden Infant Death Syndrome)
- suffocation during sleep
- car crashes
- falls

It is hard to believe that sleeping or riding in a car could hurt your baby. They are things we all do every day. Most of the time, nothing bad happens. But there is always a risk of something very serious. Every parent—and every other caregiver—needs to learn how to keep babies safe.

Look in this chapter for:

Sleep safety: SIDS and suffocation, page 214

  Safe places; Dangerous places

  Baby sleeping on his back—always

  Be careful with bed-sharing

Buckling up baby in the car, page 217

  Choosing and installing a car seat

  Buckling baby into the seat

  Getting help with using your car seat

Other ways to keep baby safe, page 222

  Preventing falls and burns

  Baby-proofing your home

  Using cloth carriers safely

Tips for partners, page 226

How can baby sleep safely?

Where baby sleeps might not be safe

Sleep is good for babies, as long as they are on their back and in a safe place. Each year, many healthy babies die in their sleep space (crib, bed, etc.). Most die from unknown reasons (SIDS*). Others die because they cannot breathe (suffocation* or strangulation*). All together, these are called "sudden unexpected infant deaths" (or SUID for short).

Of all these deaths:

◆ Most young babies (birth to 3 months) were sleeping with someone else when they died.

◆ Most older babies (4 to 12 months) had soft things in the bed with them (pillows, blankets, or toys).

Sudden infant death syndrome (SIDS)

When a healthy baby under age 1 dies in their sleep area and no one can tell why, it is called a SIDS death. This happens most to babies less than six months old. In the US, SIDS is the biggest cause of death for healthy babies in the first year of life.

It's no one's fault when a baby dies of SIDS. But, following the safe sleep advice below can help cut down on the chance of SIDS, especially in the first six months.

Suffocation and strangulation

Suffocation and strangulation happen when something keeps a baby from breathing. A baby moves a lot while sleeping. But he may not be strong enough and does not know to move his head so he can breathe. Babies can't protect themselves, so you must do it for them.

Keeping baby safe while sleeping

You can do a lot to protect your baby from sleep-related death. Be sure to do these simple things every time you put him down to sleep (at nap and at night), no matter where you are.

◆ Make the place baby sleeps as safe as possible.

◆ Put baby to sleep lying on his back.

*SIDS:
Sudden Infant Death Syndrome, sometimes called "crib death."

*Suffocation:
When a person can't breathe because something covers his nose and mouth. A baby's face might get covered if a person rolls over against him, or by a pillow or blanket. Or his head might fall forward if baby is sleeping in a baby seat.

*Strangulation:
When a person can't breathe because something is too tight around his neck. A baby might strangle in loose straps, monitor cords, or a crib bumper.

Studies show that the couch is the most dangerous place for a baby to sleep.

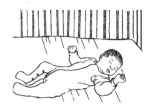

A safe place

The safest place for your baby to sleep is in a firm, flat baby bed of some kind. This might be a crib, play yard, bassinet, or cradle. Your baby's bed should meet current safety standards (see Chapter 6).

If you can't get a baby bed, use the next safest thing. A strong box, firm laundry basket, or safe place on the floor can be good choices.

A safe sleep space has:

* a firm, flat surface with no way for baby to fall off
* a mattress that fits the baby bed with no gaps at the edges where baby's head could get stuck
* no blankets, pillows, or soft toys
* no padded bumper around the edge or sleep positioner

Dangerous places for baby to sleep

* On a sofa, couch, chair, or waterbed
* In a bed with an adult, another child, or a pet
* With an adult who has been using alcohol or drugs. (Some medicines can make you sleepy enough to roll over onto your baby.)
* In other baby gear, like swings, bouncers, rockers, or car seats (except when driving). Always buckle baby in and stay where you can see him.

Think it through before putting your baby to sleep anywhere other than a baby bed. What are the risks? How can I make it as safe as possible?

Baby sleeping on his back—Always

Put your baby to bed on his back every time he sleeps, from day one. The sooner you start, the safer baby will be. He might not like it at first, but will get used to sleeping that way. Sleeping on his side or tummy can be dangerous.

Some people fear that a baby sleeping on his back could spit up and choke. For most healthy babies, this isn't true. They can breathe better and are safer on their back.

If your sleeping baby rolls over on to his tummy when he is very small, you can roll him back over. After he learns how to roll over on purpose, it's okay to let him sleep on his tummy. SIDS risk is lower by that age. Stop swaddling him

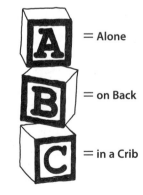

A = Alone
B = on Back
C = in a Crib

ABCs to prevent SIDS

and always put him to sleep on his back. Let him roll over on his own when he's ready.

Preemies and sick babies may need to sleep on their tummies in the hospital. Nurses or monitors are checking on them all the time to keep them safe. Most babies should start sleeping on their backs before they go home. Before you take your baby home, ask his provider if there is any medical reason for him to sleep on his tummy at home.

More important safe sleep tips

- Breastfeed your baby.
- Make sure there's no smoke (or e-cigarette vapor) near mom while she is pregnant or near baby once he's born. No smoking in the house or the car.
- Keep your baby's bed in the same room where you sleep. It is safest to have your baby in his own bed, not in yours.
- Dress him in pajamas that will keep him warm, but not hot. If he is swaddled, he may just need a onesie underneath. If he wakes up sweaty or with a red face he was too hot. Keep your heater set below 73 degrees F (23 degrees celsius).
- Give your baby a pacifier when he goes to sleep. Offer it for sleep even if he does not want one when awake. If baby has problems nursing, wait to use a pacifier until he is nursing well.
- Vaccinate your baby on time.
- Keep all cords 3 feet or more away from baby's bed. Cords on window blinds and monitors can be deadly.

Even if you can't do **all** of these things, you're still helping your baby be safer.

Be careful with bed-sharing

The safest way for baby to sleep is in his own bed, in your room. Use a bassinet, co-sleeper*, or crib next to your bed. If he falls asleep with you, you can move him to his own bed.

A baby who sleeps in bed with adults or other kids is more likely to suffocate. This could happen if someone rolls on top of him or he gets stuck against the bed or wall. But a lot of babies

*Co-sleeper: A small crib that has one low side that attaches to your bed so you can easily see and reach baby.

end up sleeping with their parents. It may seem like the only way to get baby to sleep. Or, there may not be space for a crib in the room.

It's very important to think about safety before you bring baby into bed with you, even just once. Your pillows, blankets, and even your long hair can be dangerous.

If baby does end up in your bed, try to make it safer. This can be hard. Make sure:

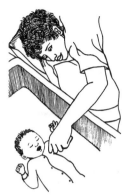

Baby's crib next to parents' bed—a safe place to sleep.

- ◆ Baby sleeps on his back, not swaddled, and is not too warm.
- ◆ There are no pillows or heavy blankets on or near him.
- ◆ The mattress is very firm.
- ◆ There is no gap at the headboard or between the bed and the wall or other furniture, where the baby's head could get stuck.
- ◆ The baby cannot fall off of the bed.
- ◆ Everyone in the bed is sober. No drugs, alcohol, or medicines that make them sleep really deeply.
- ◆ The baby does not sleep between two people.
- ◆ Your baby does not have other health problems. Healthy, full-term babies may be safer than others.

Teach your baby's caregivers about sleep safety

Make sure all people who care for your baby know they should always put him to sleep on his back. When a baby is used to sleeping on his back, SIDS can happen if he is put to sleep on his tummy just once. Tell them why soft things like blankets can be dangerous. Even when others don't agree, you get to make the rules about keeping your baby safe.

Buckling up baby for every car ride

Everyone in the car should be buckled up for every ride, even if it's short. Your baby must ride in a car seat that fits. Car seats are very good at saving lives. If his car seat is the right size and you learn how to use it right, your baby will be the safest person in the car. Car seat use is the same if baby is in a minivan, SUV, pickup truck, or taxi.

If you often take your baby in a school bus or transit bus, see page 222. Safety will be different if there are no seat belts.

Rear facing is safest until at least age 2

*Kids should ride rear facing until they are too tall or too heavy for the instructions of their car seat.

All babies and toddlers should ride rear facing. That means facing the back of the car.* Riding rear facing is safest. This is because the back of the car seat protects baby's head, neck, and back from being thrown forward. Injuries are worst to these parts of the body. Even in very bad crashes, kids riding rear facing are usually not hurt.

Kids are safest riding rear facing until they are at least 2 to 3 years old. Keep baby riding rear facing until he is too tall or too heavy for a convertible car seat's rear-facing mode.

Choosing the "best" car seat

There are a lot of car seats out there! It can be very hard to choose. There is not one best brand. The best car seat is the one that:

- has low harness (shoulder) slots to fit a new baby
- is labeled for use by babies as small as 4 to 5 pounds
- fits your car's back seat and can be buckled in tightly
- is easy to use right on every car ride

See Chapter 6 for how to choose the best car seat for you. Be sure to try it in your car before you buy it.

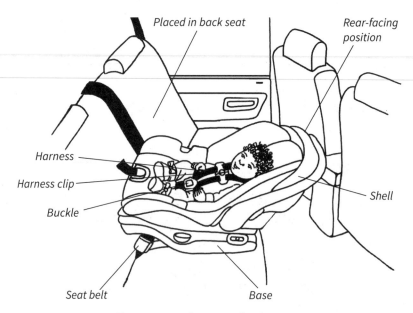

Placed in back seat

Rear-facing position

Harness

Harness clip

Buckle

Shell

Seat belt

Base

Features of car safety seats

Installing the car seat

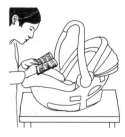

Use the middle seating position in the back seat if the car seat can be installed tightly there. If you are carrying other children or if it doesn't fit there, move it to the side.

Read the car seat booklet. It tells you what you need to know about using the car seat. Read about how to buckle it to the car and baby into the seat.

Read your car's owner's manual. Read the part that talks about installing car seats. (Car seats may be called "child restraint systems.") See if your car has LATCH* (sometimes called ISOFIX). If your car has LATCH, find out where and how you can use it. Also read how to use the seat belts to attach the car seat.

*LATCH: A way of buckling a car seat into a car instead of using a seat belt. LATCH uses special parts in the car and on the car seat. (It is sometimes called ISOFIX.)

- Where do you want baby to ride? If you want to put him in the middle of the back seat, you may need to use the seat belt. Most cars don't allow LATCH use there.

- Can you use LATCH? To use it, both the car and the car seat must have special parts that connect together. LATCH may not be usable in every seat in the car. It can only be used until your child reaches a certain weight. If your child is too heavy, use the seat belt.

- How do you lock the seat belts? There are a few kinds of seat belts. Each has a different way of being tightened around a car seat. Check the car manual.

- How far should the car seat be tipped back (reclined)? Follow the recline indicator on the side of most seats. Make sure your baby's head doesn't fall forward (picture).

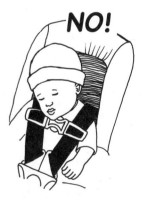

If baby's head flops forward, adjust the seat to tip back a bit more.

Most seats have a way to change the recline angle. If yours doesn't, use a rolled towel or a piece of a foam "pool noodle" under the car seat by the baby's feet to tilt it back a bit. (See picture at right.)

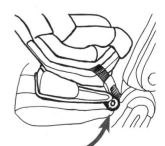

A styrofoam pool noodle can be used to tilt the car seat back.

Install the car seat tightly with the car's seat belt or LATCH. To test if it is tight, push and pull on the car seat base. The seat shouldn't move more than one inch side to side or front to back.

Air bags and babies

Never place your baby in the front seat with an air bag unless the air bag has been turned off. A baby can die if the front passenger air bag inflates. Put the car seat in front only if your car or truck has no back seat, or a very small one.

If the only place for baby to ride is in front, you must make sure the air bag is turned off. Read about it in the car manual. There will be either an air bag sensor* or a switch to turn the air bag off and on. Sensors turn the air bag off automatically. If there is a switch, you must turn off the air bag while a baby or child is riding in front. The air bag light on the dashboard tells you if the air bag is off or on. (Turn it on again when adults and teens are riding there.)

*Sensor:
An electronic device that automatically turns off the air bag when a small child is riding in the front seat. The owner's manual will tell if the car has sensors.

If you have a really old car and aren't sure it has a front passenger air bag, look for a warning label on the sun visor. The car owner's manual will have details about air bags if it has them.

Buckling your baby into the car seat

1. The crotch strap must go between his legs.
2. Shoulder straps should come out of the seat at baby's shoulder or a bit lower. It is not safe for them to be higher than that.
3. The harness must be snug. To test it, pinch the strap between your fingers (see picture). If you can pinch any slack, it is not snug enough.
4. Put the chest clip so it points to your baby's armpits.

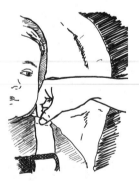

Pinch the strap to see if it is too loose. This one needs to be tightened.

Helpful car seat tips

♦ Many car seats come with pads to help baby sit without flopping. If not, you can put rolled blankets or cloth diapers next to your baby on both sides, from his hip to his head (see picture on the next page). Don't put anything under or behind him, unless it came with the seat.

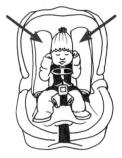

- There are lots of pads and other things sold for use with car seats. Don't use any of these unless they come from the car seat company.

- Dress your baby in clothes with legs. This allows the buckle to go between his legs. Avoid dresses, gowns, and sacks. Never wrap or swaddle your baby before putting him into the car seat.

- In cold weather, put your baby in thin fleece or wool pants or pajamas. Do not use a padded snowsuit or bunting. After he's buckled in and the straps are snug, you can cover him with a blanket. Tuck it around his arms and legs. Remember to take blankets off as the car warms up so baby doesn't get too warm.

Pad the sides of the car seat with small rolled blankets or towels (arrows). Add a rolled washcloth between his legs if there's extra space behind the crotch strap.

Getting help with using your car seat

Car seats can be confusing. Most car seats are used wrong in some ways. Have your car seat checked by a certified Child Passenger Safety Technician. Find a trained technician or a car seat checkup (or inspection station) near you. These are listed at the SeatCheck website or phone line (see Chapter 17). Checkups are very helpful and usually free.

"My friend gave me a puffy snowsuit. It was so thick I couldn't get the car seat harness tight. So I only use it in the stroller."

Car beds for babies with breathing problems

Some babies have medical problems and need to lie flat. These babies may have to ride in a special car bed. Babies who are born very early may breathe better flat on their back for a few weeks. Other babies may need to ride lying down for longer because of health issues. If your baby needs a car bed, ask your nurse or Child Passenger Safety Technician to help you get one.

All preemies born before 37 weeks should be tested sitting in his car seat before leaving the hospital. This is to make sure he can breathe well sitting up. If the baby has any trouble breathing, he should ride lying flat for a few weeks. (He also should not sit in a swing or baby seat at home until he is older.) If your baby was born early, ask his provider about "apnea testing" in a car seat.

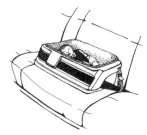

This car bed is mainly for preemies.

Car seats in taxis and school or transit buses

Use a car seat in any vehicle with seat belts, like a taxi. Do it the same way as you do in a regular car.

If you are a teen, you may take your baby with you in a school bus. In some places buses have seat belts. You may be able to use a small rear-facing car seat. Ask your driver if the district provides car seats.

In buses (or trains) without seat belts, there's no really safe way to carry baby. Sit with baby in a seat that faces forward, not the side of the bus. A car seat with a handle might give some protection even if it's not buckled in. Always use baby's harness in the seat. You could wear baby in a carrier. That would allow your hands to be free for holding on.

Never leave baby alone in a car!

Babies die every year from being left alone in a parked car. A parked car can turn into an oven quickly. Even if it's not hot outside, the car can get really hot in just a few minutes. Cracking a window or parking in the shade doesn't help.

Some babies are left in the car to nap. Some drivers just want to make a quick stop but get delayed. This is a kind of child neglect.

Sometimes babies are forgotten in the car by tired or stressed parents or other caregivers. Here are ways to prevent leaving baby in the car.

*   Make a habit of putting your bag or backpack on the floor of the back seat. This will make you look in back when you get out.

*   If your baby goes to child care, ask the caregiver to call if baby isn't there by a certain time.

Other ways to keep baby safe
Preventing falls

Babies are often wiggly and hard to hold onto. When you are busy or tired, it is easy to drop baby.

Try not to do too many things at once while holding baby. Use a carrier to wear baby when you need a free hand. (Make sure you use the carrier right, pages 225.) If you have a lot to

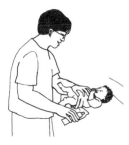

Keep one hand on baby.

put things into a backpack. If you have tasks to do, put baby in a safe place until you are done. Safe places for baby would be:

◆ A crib or play yard

◆ A clean space on the floor with a blanket under him.

A lively baby can slip off of a bed or table. When you change, bathe, or dress your baby, always keep one hand on his body. Have everything you need where you can reach it before you start.

Other things you can do to keep baby safe from falls:

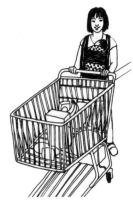

Shopping is a great time to wear your baby.

◆ Never leave him alone on a chair, table, bed, or counter, even for a second.

◆ Always buckle safety straps on baby gear.

◆ If baby is in a car seat or bouncy seat, don't put it on top of anything tall. Put it on the floor instead.

◆ Don't put baby's car seat on top of a shopping cart. If you do bring baby's seat into the store, put it in the big part of the cart. Wearing your baby leaves your hands free and keeps baby safe.

◆ Put strong baby gates at the top and bottom of the stairs before baby learns to crawl. Keep them closed. Make sure a gate is made for use on stairs. Some are not strong enough. Get a gate you can open with one hand.

◆ Don't put cribs or other furniture near windows. Use window locks to keep windows from opening more than 4 inches. That keeps a baby from falling out.

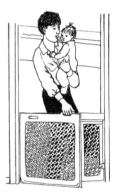

Use a gate you can open with one hand.

Preventing burns

Your baby's skin is very thin and can burn easily. Here are ways to prevent burns:

◆ **Bath temperature:** Make sure the bath water is just barely warm. Test it with your elbow. Turn down the temperature of your hot water heater to 120 degrees.

◆ **Hot things around the house:** A curling iron, hot pan, or an iron can fall on and burn a baby. Push them to the back of counters and put away cords where baby can't reach them.

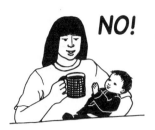

NO!

Don't drink hot liquids with baby in your lap.

- **Hot liquids:** Don't hold a hot drink or eat hot soup while you hold your baby. He could reach for it or bump it so it spills. Don't use the stove or microwave while holding baby, even in a carrier. Try to eat, drink, and cook while he is playing or sleeping.

- **Things heated by the sun:** Things sitting in the sun can get too hot for baby's skin. Cover baby's car seat when it's left in the car. Always touch benches or swings before putting baby on them when you're out and about.

- **Sunburn:** When your baby is outside during the day, keep him mostly in the shade. Dress him in light clothes that cover his arms and legs. If you can't, use a bit of baby sunscreen. (See Chapter 11.)

Baby-proofing your house now

Start making your home safe before baby starts moving on his own. Many ordinary things in your home could cause injuries. Taking care of them now means fewer things you have to worry about every day.

Smoke alarms and carbon monoxide detectors

Smoke alarms can save your whole family from a house fire. Make sure you have at least one on each floor of your home. They are especially needed outside the bedrooms.

Carbon monoxide (CO) detectors can save your family from gas poisoning. CO is a deadly gas that you can't see or smell. CO detectors are needed if you have a gas stove or furnace, oil heat, or any kind of fireplace. Put one on each level of your home. If you can, put them below waist height.

Test all alarms often. Change the batteries at least once a year or put in 10-year batteries. Pick a day you will remember each year, like the day you turn the clocks ahead in spring.

Dangers as babies learn to crawl and climb

"My doctor said that if I don't trust baby to be alone with something for 10 seconds, then keep it out of reach."

As your baby learns to crawl, stand, and climb, he is more likely to fall. Put gates up to keep him away from stairs. There are also many dangerous things he could get into. The best way to protect your baby is to keep those things where he can't see or reach. Get down on hands and knees for a baby's-eye view of your home.

- **Poisons and medicines:** Put all of your cleaners in a high cabinet and put a lock on it. Do the same with all of your medicines and vitamins. **Put Poison Control's phone number by all of your phones: 1-800-222-1222.**

- **Sharp things:** Keep knives and scissors out of reach.

- **Electric sockets and cords:** Put covers on electric outlets and put cords out of sight and reach. Tie up cords of curtains and window shades.

- **Heaters:** Put baby gates around the fireplace, wood stove, and heaters.

- **Guns:** Lock guns or other weapons in a gun safe.

Having dangerous things put out of reach or locked up makes caring for baby easier. It's more fun than saying "no" and taking things away all the time.

Babies will put anything in their mouths to learn about them. Sweep or vacuum the floor often. If you have pets, make sure their litter boxes, food, and water dishes are kept away from baby.

Babies like to pull themselves up when learning to walk. Some start climbing very early. Heavy things can tip over onto a baby. Bolt tall furniture like book shelves and dressers to the wall. Attach your TV to the wall so it can't fall.

No place is ever completely baby-proof. As baby grows, watch out for new risks around the house and yard. Make sure that other homes where your baby spends time are also baby-proofed. When you visit other places, watch baby closely just in case things are not as safe there.

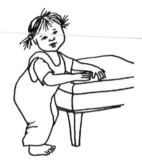

Soon your baby will be able get into things that you thought were out of reach.

Using other gear safely

Using a cloth baby carrier

When you wear your baby in a carrier or sling, remember these safety tips, called TICKS:

T—Tight, hugging baby to your body

I—In view, where you can see her face easily

C—Close enough to give baby a kiss

K—Keep baby's neck straight, not flopped forward or back

S—Support baby's back so she doesn't curl up and her chin doesn't fall onto her chest.

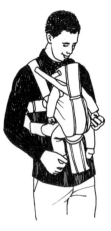

A carrier with straps keeps baby's head from flopping.

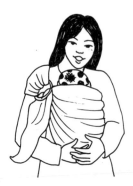

Keep baby upright in a sling.

Learn how to put baby into your carrier with a friend helping to make sure baby doesn't fall. Or, try it sitting on your bed, just in case. After you get baby in, look in a mirror and go through the TICKS checklist above. Make sure to read all instructions for your carrier.

If you have a used carrier, check it for recalls. Make sure it is in good shape with no holes, tears, or loose threads. See Chapter 17 for where to learn more about wearing your baby.

Second-hand baby gear

Using gently used baby gear can save a lot of money. Avoid used car seats unless you know it hasn't been in a crash (Chapter 6). For car seats and other gear, make sure you have the instructions so you can use it correctly. Check to see that all of the parts are there and put together well. Look to see if it has been recalled.

Steer clear of old plastic baby seats

You might find one of these at a garage sale or in your parents' attic. These look a lot like car seats but are light and have thin straps. There is no way to use them safely. It's best to throw one in the trash if you find it. Take out the straps and pad first, so no one else will try to use it.

Tips for partners

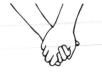

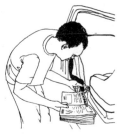

Use the vehicle and car seat manuals to use baby's car seat right.

- ◆ Have baby sleep in his own bed, in your room. Talk to your partner about how you can help at night.
- ◆ Learn how to use your baby's car seat right: rear facing with a snug harness. Make sure to follow the directions. Go to a car seat checkup with your partner.
- ◆ Learn the pinch test for car seat harness tightness. If you can squeeze a fold in the strap, it's too loose.
- ◆ Help with babyproofing. Make sure to close gates at the top and bottom of the stairs.
- ◆ Put all small things up high. Coins, keys, batteries, and other small things are dangerous for baby.
- ◆ Help keep the floors clean.
- ◆ Got your hands full? Wear baby in a carrier.

Chapter 15

Keeping Your Baby Healthy

Good health care is more than what your baby's doctor or nurse does. You, your partner, and her provider are a team. Here are four ways you lead the team.

1. Take your baby for all of her checkups.

2. Make sure she gets vaccines on time.

3. Learn to tell if she is sick and when to call her provider.

4. Learn ways to care for your sick baby at home.

5. Provide a healthy home and take the steps to protect baby from illness and from injury.

Look in this chapter for:

Ways to keep baby healthy, page 228

How to wash your hands well

Your baby's well-baby checkups, page 229

Why healthy babies need checkups

Vaccines fight deadly diseases, page 230

Why babies need vaccines on time

When your baby gets sick, page 235

Warning signs—First few months, page 236

Taking your baby's temperature

Giving medicine to a baby

Taking care of baby teeth, page 239

Tips for partners, page 240

Your baby's first checkups, page 241

Ways to Keep Baby Healthy

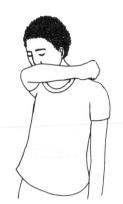

Cough into your arm or sleeve. This prevents hands from getting covered with germs and passing them on.

- Breastfeed your baby so she gets antibodies from you to fight germs.
- Wash your hands often and make sure others do, too. If you can't wash, use hand sanitizer.
- Keep her away from people who are smoking. Ask people who smoke to do it outside and wash their hands afterwards.
- If you cough or sneeze, cover your nose and mouth with your sleeve or arm, not your hand.
- Keep your baby away from people who have colds, coughs, fevers, or other sickness. They may not seem very sick. But they could spread germs that are dangerous for babies.
- Avoid taking her into crowds, like malls and movie theaters, for the first few months.

Hand washing—An easy way to protect baby

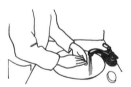

Make hand washing a habit. Make sure everyone who cares for your baby washes their hands with soap often. This is the best way to keep germs from spreading.

- Wash your hands before feeding, touching or playing with your baby, or mixing formula for a bottle.
- Wash hands after using the bathroom, changing her diaper, handling raw foods, blowing your nose, or caring for pets.
- Wash hands more often if you are sick.
- Wash after going to the store or getting gas.
- Make sure older kids wash after coming home from school or playing outside. They should not touch the baby if they are sick.
- Wash your baby's hands before she eats or goes to bed. Wash after she plays on the floor. Wash if she puts her hands near her bottom during a diaper change.

> ### How to Wash Your Hands Well
>
> 1. Use warm water and regular soap.
> 2. Rub soapy hands together for 15 to 20 seconds (the time it takes to hum the "Happy Birthday" song slowly). It can take that long to get the germs out of finger nails and creases.
> 3. Rinse and dry with a clean towel.

Use hand sanitizers, not "anti-bacterial" soaps

If you can't wash with plain soap and water every time, use a hand sanitizer without water. Hand gels and sprays are made with alcohol. They do a good job of killing most germs.

Don't use any cleaners that say they are anti-bacterial. First, they do **not** kill the viruses that cause most sickness. Also, these cleaners can lead to growth of super-germs that antibiotics can't fight. That means if you get sick later on, antibiotics may not help.

Your baby's well-baby checkups

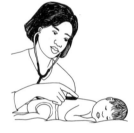

Your baby's doctor will want to see her for her first checkup when she is 2 to 5 days old. After that, well-baby checkups are at 2 weeks, 4 weeks, then at 2, 4, 6, 9, and 12 months.

Why does a healthy baby need to see a provider?

Well-baby checkups help keep your baby healthy. The doctor or nurse will check her body, growth, and development.

He may spot problems that you can't see. Finding problems early can keep them from getting serious. He will make sure you don't worry more than you need to.

What happens at a well-baby checkup?

At each checkup, the doctor or nurse will weigh your baby and measure her length and head size. He will check ears, eyes, mouth, lungs, heart, abdomen, penis or vagina, hips, legs, and reflexes.

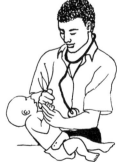

Your baby will get vaccines at most checkups. Different vaccines are given at different ages. (See schedule, page 234.)

The provider will check your baby's development. He will look for the things she is learning to do, such as holding up her head

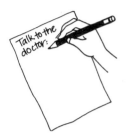

Use the notes page at the end of this chapter to keep track of your baby's early checkups and first vaccines.

and smiling. Be sure to tell him the new things that you have seen your baby do. You know your baby best. If you think she isn't developing, tell the doctor that, too.

Asking questions

Checkups are the best time to ask the doctor or nurse any questions you have. Bring a list of things you want to talk about to the checkup. Write down what the provider tells you, so you can remember later.

Baby's record of vaccines (immunizations or shots)

Your clinic or health department will give you a card to keep a record of your baby's checkups and vaccines. You will need this information if you change doctors. When your child goes to child care or school, you will need to know the vaccines she has had. Keep the card in a safe place. Bring it to all your baby's checkups.

Vaccines fight deadly diseases
Why do babies need vaccines

Your baby needs vaccines to protect her from some very serious diseases like measles, diphtheria, polio, and tetanus. These diseases spread easily from person to person. Before vaccines were discovered, many people died from these diseases. Many more people were left with lifelong disabilities like deafness or trouble walking.

Vaccines are made from the germs that cause these diseases. When your baby gets a vaccine, her body makes cells to fight off those germs. These cells make her immune to (very unlikely to catch) those diseases. Thanks to vaccines, many of these diseases hardly ever happen today. Because of this, many people don't know how serious they can be.

*Outbreak:
When a people in an area catch one disease from each other.

Even today, outbreaks* can happen, such as with measles or pertussis (whooping cough). The illness can be caused by a person who never got the vaccine. He may carry the germs but not know he's sick. Then a baby who isn't vaccinated can catch the germs.

Outbreaks of Measles Really Happen

In 2014 there was a big outbreak of measles in the U.S. Another outbreak in January 2015 started at a crowded amusement park. Children who got sick had not had the MMR vaccine. Schoolmates who also had not had that vaccine had to stay home from school for 21 days.

Measles isn't just a mild sickness with cough and an itchy rash. It can cause many dangerous effects, even death. It can spread four days before a person starts to feel sick. Babies can't get the MMR vaccine until they are a year old so lots of babies and others are in danger.

Measles isn't the only disease a baby can catch in the U.S. Babies and others with weak immune systems are safe only when most everyone has had all required vaccines.

Once someone gets sick, their germs spread easily to others who haven't had the vaccine. This is especially dangerous for:

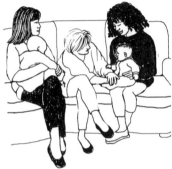

- ◆ Babies too young to get vaccines that are usually given at 6 or 12 months

- ◆ Children whose parents decided not to give vaccines to them

- ◆ People with weak immune systems whose bodies can't fight diseases well

So, giving your baby all vaccines for her age helps protect her and everyone else.

Unfortunately, there is no vaccine for the common cold. So keep new babies away from crowds and people who are coughing and sneezing and have sore throats.

"I was glad to get my baby immunized. Now I don't have to worry that someone might pass a serious illness to my child."

Get vaccines on time

It's important to get your baby immunized as soon as possible. Don't wait until your child goes to child care or school.

There are 10 vaccines made to prevent 14 diseases as of 2014. Some are combined so fewer shots are needed. Babies need more than one dose of most vaccines for full protection.

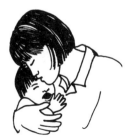

Older kids and adults have to get booster shots of some vaccines to stay immune. Flu vaccine is different. It must be given to everyone each year because the flu germs change each year.

Vaccines and the Diseases They Prevent

Many of these diseases are rare today. Before vaccines were invented, they were very serious. Most spread through the air, by coughing, sneezing, or just breathing. Some are spread by dirty hands or blood from a person who has the germs.

DTaP, for diphtheria, tetanus, and pertussis.

> **Diphtheria** (dif-thee-ree-a) can cause heart and breathing problems, paralysis, or death. It is spread through the air.

> **Tetanus** (lockjaw) causes severe muscle and breathing problems and, often, death. It spreads through cuts in the skin.

> **Pertussis** (whooping cough) can cause severe coughing, lung problems, seizures, brain damage, or death in babies. It is spread through the air. (An adult or older child with a cough may have pertussis but not feel sick.)

HepA for hepatitis A, a liver disease spreads by stool (poop) in dirty food or water or on hands.

HepB for hepatitis B, another liver disease. It spreads in blood or spit and can pass from mother to baby.

Hib for haemophilus influenzae b (hay-ma-fill-us in-flew-en-zay b), which causes meningitis (brain swelling) and can lead to brain damage or death. It is spread in the air.

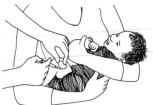

Babies often are given shots in their thighs.

You may not like seeing your baby get so many shots. Remember that it only hurts her for a little while and it will protect her for many years. To comfort your baby, speak softly, cuddle her, show her a toy, or nurse her.

No vaccine works 100 percent of the time. Sometimes people get a disease even though they have been vaccinated, but they usually don't get very sick. Booster shots help keep children's immunity high. Talk with your baby's doctor or nurse if you have questions about immunizing your baby.

You may hear about an outbreak in your community that puts your baby in danger. Check with her provider about giving her a dose of some vaccines early to protect her.

Influenza for "the flu" that comes every winter. It can be deadly for babies and elders. It spreads through the air.

MMR for measles, mumps, and rubella.

Measles can cause deafness, brain damage, pneumonia (new-mo-nee-ah), or death. It is spread through the air.

Mumps can cause convulsions, deafness, brain damage, or death. It spreads by coughing, sneezing, breathing.

Rubella (German measles) can cause mild sickness in kids. But, if a pregnant woman gets rubella, her baby may be born deaf or blind, or have brain or heart damage. She may also have a miscarriage. It spreads through the air.

PCV for pneumococcal (new-mo-cock-al) disease, which can cause swelling of the brain and spinal cord, blood or lung infections, or death. It spreads through the air.

Polio (IPV) for polio, which can cause life-long paralysis or death. It is spread by stool (poop) on hands or in water.

RV for rotavirus, which can cause severe vomiting and diarrhea. This leads to loss of a large amount of water. That can cause death. It is spread through stool.

Varicella for chickenpox, which can cause skin rash and brain swelling. Chickenpox can be deadly for babies, even if they are not born yet. It is spread through the air or by touching the rash.

Common questions about vaccines

Learning the truth about vaccines can be confusing. A lot of scary things you hear about them on the Internet or in the news are not true. Check the vaccine resources in Chapter 17 for the facts about common worries.

Can my baby get vaccines even when she has a cold? It is almost always OK for your baby to get vaccines when she is mildly sick. But, it's good to tell her provider she's sick first.

What if we miss a well-baby checkup? Make another appointment and go in soon so you can keep your baby's immunizations up-to-date.

What side effects could my baby have after vaccines? Some will give your baby no side effects. Others may make your baby's arm or leg red or puffy where the shot was given. She may get a

Vaccines Recommended by Age 2 as of 2015

Age when usually given	Vaccine name
Birth	HepB
2 months	HepB (1–2 months), DTaP, PCV, Hib, Polio, RV
4 months	DTaP, PCV, Hib, Polio, RV
6 months	HepB (6–18 months), DTaP, PCV, Hib, Polio (6–36 mos), RV
12–15 months	MMR, PCV, Hib, Varicella, HepA (12-23 months)
15–18 months	DTaP
Other vaccines	**Range of months when it can be given**
Influenza (flu)	Babies 6 months and older should get 1–2 doses each Fall or Winter

Other vaccines or boosters will be given to school-age children and teens.

Special shots may be needed if your baby is bitten by an animal or travels to other parts of the world where other diseases are common.

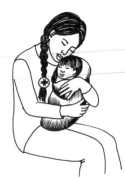

fever or be fussy for a few days. Ask the doctor or nurse how to comfort your baby and what reactions you should call about.

Is it bad for baby to get so many vaccines at one time? No, but it can be hard for parents to watch. Each shot does hurt for a short time after it's given.

Can a baby get really sick from a vaccine? It is very, very rare for a baby to have a severe reaction. Rumors about problems caused by vaccines have been found to be not true. However, if your baby seems to be sick after getting a vaccine, be sure to call the doctor or nurse.

If I do not want my child to get a vaccine required for child care or school, can she still go? Each state has different laws. In many states, a child who is not immunized can go if parents sign a state waiver form. If an outbreak of disease happens, the child would have to stay home until it's over.

Not being immunized could be dangerous for your child and others. Parents must understand that a child who does not get all her vaccines could catch a serious, preventable illness. She also could spread that illness to others easily.

When Your Baby Gets Sick

If your baby looks or behaves differently than normal

You will soon learn what is normal for her. Many babies don't get sick in the first three months. If you are worried, it is best to talk with her doctor or nurse. If your health plan or provider has a phone number for medical advice, you could call it. Providers expect new parents to call as often as they need to.

The only silly questions are the ones you don't ask.

Nights and weekends, if you cannot reach your doctor or nurse, call an urgent care center or after-hours clinic. If it seems serious, take your baby to an emergency room. If you think your baby's life could be in danger, call 9-1-1.

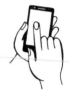

Two baby illnesses to know about

- **Newborn Jaundice:** Too much bilirubin in the blood that makes a new baby's skin turn yellow. Most jaundice is mild and goes away soon. If you are breastfeeding, nurse baby as often as possible in the first few days. If it gets worse (or your baby's eyes and hands look yellow) between newborn checkups, call the doctor or nurse. Serious jaundice can lead to brain damage if it is not treated.

- **RSV:** A virus that starts like a cold but gets much worse quickly. Baby's lungs could fill with mucus, making it very hard for her to breathe. Call the doctor right away if she has a fever, thick green or gray mucus from her nose, heavy breathing, wheezing, or a cough. (It is easy to catch RSV from crowds of people or things a sick person has touched.)

Fever: Taking your baby's temperature

If your baby has a fever, it means her body is fighting off an illness.

Any fever in a baby younger than 2 months old could be serious. If you think she has one, call her provider right away. But first, take her temperature. You can't know your baby has a fever just by feeling her forehead.

Warning Signs—First Few Months

Any of these signs could mean your baby is very sick. Call right away if your baby has:

- **Yellow skin or eyes** (jaundice), most likely in the first 2 to 3 weeks.

- **Infection** of the umbilical cord or circumcised penis: pus* or bright red blood and a red area around the cord stump or tip of the penis.

  > ***Pus:** Gooey, smelly, white or yellow discharge from an infected cut.

- **Temperature** under about 97° F or over 99° F (when taken in the armpit) or over 100.4° (taken rectally). Always use a thermometer, not your hands, to decide if your baby has a fever.

- **No appetite**: if baby doesnt want the breast or bottle for two feedings in a row.

- **No wet diapers** in 12 hours or less than 6 wet diapers in 24 hours. (It can be hard to tell if a disposible diaper is wet. Putting a tissue inside it helps you know if it gets wet.)

- **Bloody poops or none at all, or very hard ones.**

- **Vomiting with force** (shooting 2 or 3 feet out of baby's mouth) or for more than 6 hours.

- **Diarrhea** (die-ah-ree-ah): two or more poops that are smelly and watery (and often green), or more than 8 soft stools in 24 hours.

- **Hard tummy** that feels very full.

- **Thick yellow-green mucus** in baby's nose.

- **Oozing liquid or blood** coming from any opening. (Tiny drops of milk from baby's breasts or blood from the vagina are normal in the first week.)

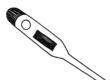

Digital thermometer

There are several kinds of thermometers that you can use for a baby. The most common and cheapest is digital. Others are for use on the forehead or in the ear. Forehead strips, and pacifier thermometers do not give a true temperature. (Old-fashioned glass thermometers should not be used.)

There are four ways to take a baby's temperature. They give different readings for a fever. Practice taking your baby's

- ◆ **Breathing problems:**
  - ▪ **Breathing too fast**—more than 60 breaths per minute (babies normally breathe much faster than adults do)
  - ▪ **Very heavy breathing**, having a hard time breathing (baby's skin pulls in around the ribs when she breathes)
  - ▪ **Flared nostrils (open wide), wheezing, grunting**
  - ▪ **No breaths** for more than 15 seconds
  - ▪ **Coughing** that doesn't go away or makes it hard for baby to breathe
- ◆ **Bluish skin**, lips, tongue, or white toes and fingertips (except when baby is cold or crying hard)
- ◆ **More crying** than usual, especially high-pitched shrieks
- ◆ **Sleepier** than usual, little movement, very floppy body
- ◆ **Jittery** or shaky movements
- ◆ **Hearing problem** if baby does not notice loud noises

It's always better to call than to just worry.

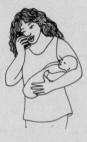

Before calling the doctor

- ◆ Take your baby's temperature if you think she may have a fever. Write down how high it is, how you took it, and at what time.
- ◆ Write down what is making you worry (for example: pale skin, screaming cry, no stools, vomiting, or diarrhea).
- ◆ Have a pencil and paper ready when you call. Use these to write down what the doctor or nurse tells you.

Call your provider's office or a consulting nurse. They will tell you what you can do at home to help your baby feel better. They may ask you to bring your baby into the office or go to an urgent-care clinic or emergency room.

temperature when she is not sick. This will give you an idea of what her normal temperature is. The different ways are:

- ◆ **In the bottom** (rectal) with a digital thermometer. It gives the best reading for kids under age 3. 100.4° F or higher is a fever and you should call your baby's provider.
- ◆ **In the armpit** (axillary) which is not very accurate, but good for a quick check. Use a digital thermometer. With

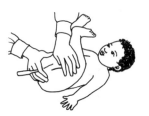

Taking rectal
temperature
in baby's bottom

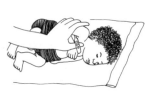

Taking baby's
temperature
in the armpit

Forehead (temporal
artery) thermometer

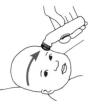

Ear (tympanic)
thermometer

this method, 99° F is a fever and you should take it again rectally or call baby's provider.

- **Across the forehead** (temporal artery), using a special thermometer, is good for babies under 3 months old. A fever is 100.4° F or higher.

- **In the ear** (tympanic), using a special thermometer, only for babies older than 6 months. A fever is 100.4° F or higher.

Ask your health care provider which way she thinks is best. Ask how high it should be before you call. When you report baby's temperature, be sure to tell which way you took it.

The armpit is often the easiest place to take a baby's temperature. It works to get a basic temperature, but rectal is better for an exact reading.

In the armpit: Lift your baby's arm and put the tip of the digital thermometer into her armpit. Lower her arm and hold it down against her body until the thermometer beeps.

In the bottom (rectal): Put a bit of petroleum jelly on the end of a clean digital thermometer. Lay baby on her back to keep her still. Bend her knees to her chest with your hand on the back of her thighs to keep her still. Gently put the tip of the thermometer into her bottom 1/2 to 1 inch. Going in too far will hurt her. Gently pull the thermometer out when it beeps.

Giving medicine to a baby

Most of the time, a baby with a fever will be just fine without medicine. Fevers help her body fight off germs. But, if a fever gets too high (see warning signs) or baby is having a hard time, it may be time for some baby medicine.

Before giving any kind of medicine to your baby, ask her doctor or nurse. Make sure the medicine is safe for your baby's age and size. Some medicine, like aspirin or cough syrup, should never be given to a baby. Other medicines, like ibuprofen, should not be given until she's at least 6 months old.

Make sure you follow the directions to give the right amount of medicine. This usually depends on the baby's weight and age.

Most baby medicine is a liquid. Use the dropper or medicine syringe (sir-INJ) that comes with it. If you don't have one, you can ask for one at the drug store. Follow the directions to measure carefully. Squirt the medicine in the side of baby's mouth, between her tongue and cheek.

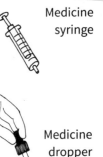

Medicine syringe

Medicine dropper

Some medicine comes as a suppository, which is like a pill that goes into baby's bottom. The medicine melts into baby's body. This is easier than swallowing liquid.

Warnings about giving antibiotics

An antibiotic drug is only useful for certain kinds of illness. If the doctor prescribes one, be sure to give it to baby as long as it says on the bottle. Stopping it too soon may make it work less well the next time your baby needs it.

Use antibiotics only for what the doctor prescribes them for. They do not help colds or the flu. Using an antibiotic when it is **not** needed is not good for baby or for you.

Keep track of your baby's checkups and immunizations on the last page of the chapter.

Follow directions for storing medicines. Some need to be kept in the refrigerator. Store all drugs out of reach of children.

Taking care of baby teeth

It is important to keep baby teeth healthy. Your baby needs those teeth for many things besides chewing food. Teeth help baby talk. They also hold space in the gums for her second set of teeth.

When her first teeth start coming in, wipe them daily or use a soft baby toothbrush. If you use any toothpaste, use only a tiny smear (like a grain of rice) on the brush. Ask your baby's doctor or nurse if you should use toothpaste with fluoride.

Tips for partners

- Help make sure your baby gets to all of her checkups. Go to checkups when you can. It is the best way for you to know what baby's provider says.

- Make sure your own vaccines are up to date. Take care of yourself so you don't get sick. Young babies often get germs from their parents or other caregivers.

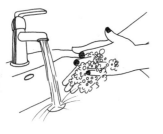

- Wash your hands often. Use soap. Scrub front and back, between fingers and under nails.

- If you have been around a sick person or anything dirty, change your clothes before you hold baby.

- Limit guests. Don't invite anyone who may be sick to visit while baby is new.

- Learn the warning signs (earlier in this chapter) so you know how to tell when your baby is sick.

- Make sure the 24-hour phone number for her doctor or nurse is in your phone.

- Know where the nearest urgent care clinic or emergency room is.

Your baby's first checkups

Newborn screening

____ First blood screen (before going home)

____ Second blood screen (if required in your state) in the second week

Comments: _____

_____

Remember: follow up on any screens that show the need for other tests.

Well-baby checkups

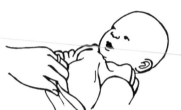

(The exact schedule will depend on your baby's health and on your health care provider or insurance plan.)

Questions you may want to ask at the next checkup:

How does my baby's height and weight compare with that of other babies? or *What percentile is my baby in?*

_____

_____

_____

First checkup (1 to 2 weeks) (date) _____

Baby's age _____ weeks; weight _____ pounds, _____ ounces;

Length _____ inches; head size _____ inches

Comments: _____

Date and time of next checkup: _____

Questions you may want to ask at the next checkup:

Does my baby need extra Vitamin D or fluoride?

How is my baby developing?

_____

_____

_____

Second checkup (2 months) (date) _____

Baby's age _____ weeks; weight _____ pounds, _____ ounces;

Length _____ inches; head size _____ inches

Comments: _____

_____

Date and time of next checkup
(usually at 4 months): _____

First vaccines baby has been given

First doses of vaccines   **Dates given**

Hep B: first at birth to 2 months   _____

DTP: first at 2 months   _____

Polio: first at 2 months   _____

Hib: first at 2 months   _____

RV: first at 2 months   _____

Keep a permanent, long-term record of vaccines or immunizations on a form from your doctor or nurse or clinic. You will need it to show child care and school district the shots that baby has had.

Chapter 16

Taking Care of Yourself

Remember to take care of your own health! Your body and mind need to recover from giving birth so you can take good care of your baby.

For the first few weeks after birth, you need plenty of rest and time to get to know your baby. It's okay if all you want to do now is eat, sleep, and care for your baby. Those are your most important jobs right now. Of course, if you have other young kids, also spend at least a little time with them.

Let your family and friends help out now. You may need to tell them what would be most helpful. Sometimes a person wants to help but makes you feel stressed out. Ask them to do things out of the house. Ideas would be walking the dog, doing food shopping, or cooking food to bring over.

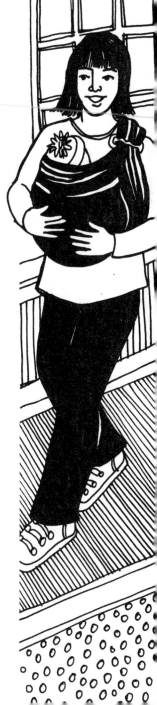

Look in this chapter for:

What to expect as your body heals, page 244

Warning signs—The first few weeks, page 245

   Keep up your healthy habits

Your own six-week checkup, page 248

Sex after baby, page 248

How Are You Feeling?, page 250

   Mood disorders after giving birth

   Is it more than just baby blues?

   What to do

Tips for partners, page 253

Affirmations for parents, page 254

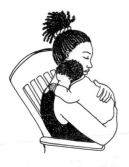

Keeping the stress down at home

Don't worry too much about house work. Just let the dust pile up for a while. Let other people help with things like laundry, making dinner, doing the dishes, and cleaning the bathroom. They could hold baby while you take a shower and eat.

It's nice to have loved ones come to visit, but let them know to keep it short. You should feel OK about saying that it's time for you and baby to take a nap. Don't feel like you need to entertain people or take care of others right now. It is also okay to say "no visitors today" or ask people to leave meals or gifts outside the door.

A home visit from a nurse

Some health programs or clinics may offer a visit from a nurse a few days after you get home. Ask your provider about this. If you can get it, it is a wonderful service. A nurse would come to see how you both are doing. She would answer questions about your baby's needs and your recovery. She could give you hands-on help with baby care and breastfeeding.

What to expect as your body heals

- ◆ **Birth can make you very tired.** You may ache or feel sore. Talk to your doctor or midwife about pain medicine that is safe for you now. Taking it on time will help you rest and heal.

- ◆ **You will have discharge** from your vagina for a few weeks. Use pads only, not tampons. At first, it will be heavy and bright red, and may have clots (thick blobs). Then, it should slow down and turn pink or brown.

- ◆ **If the discharge** turns bright red again, you should rest more. If the bleeding gets heavier, see warning signs on the next page, then call your doctor or midwife right away.

- ◆ **Your uterus will start to shrink.** Use the Kegel squeeze and the pelvic tilt (page 21) to help your vagina and tummy get back in shape.

- ◆ **You may have cramps,** especially when you are nursing. If they get very painful, call your doctor or nurse.

Warning Signs—The First Few Weeks

Call your provider if you have:

- Heavy bleeding—blood clots bigger than an egg or bright red blood that soaks your menstrual pad in an hour or less.
- Discharge from your vagina that smells bad.
- Fever or flu-like symptoms.
- Trouble urinating or having bowel movements.
- Pain near or in your vagina, bottom, or belly.
- Signs of infection (pus, redness, soreness, or swelling) from your stitches (from a c-section, episiotomy, or tear).
- Pain in your breasts; breast that have warm areas; nipples that are cracked or very sore.
- Swelling in one or both legs, or a warm, painful area in one leg.
- Feeling very emotional or sad. Having trouble sleeping. See the section of moods later in this chapter.

- **If you had an episiotomy or tear,** you will be sore. Keep the area clean. Change your pad often. Soak in a very shallow (sitz) bath or use witch hazel pads (from the drug store) or cold packs. Make cold packs by soaking maxi pads in water or witch hazel and cooling them in the freezer.

- **Eating foods with fiber helps to prevent constipation.** There is lots of fiber in fresh fruits and vegetables, bran cereal, and dried apricots or prunes. Also, drink at least 8 to 10 glasses of water a day. Your doctor or midwife may also advise using stool softener pills.

- **If you had a tear or stitches from an episiotomy,** sitting down or going to the bathroom may be painful. Hard chairs may be easier for sitting. When sitting down on the toilet, squeeze your cheeks (buttocks) together, then sit. Spread your legs to both sides of the toilet for more comfort.

"I tried eating lots of fruits and veggies but I was still constipated. When I started drinking lots of water, too, it worked better. Prune juice worked really well."

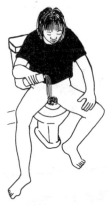

Squirt warm water around your vagina to make peeing easier.

- **If it's hard to pee (urinate),** drink lots of water. Try to pee when you are in the shower. While sitting on the toilet, squirt warm water on the area. If pee doesn't come out, call your doctor or midwife.

- **While pooping (pushing stool out),** hold some toilet paper or a witch hazel pad against the stitches and press up to protect the stitches. Wipe from front to back and clean your bottom carefully.

- **Put nothing into your vagina for at least 6 weeks.** That means no sex or tampons. Don't forget to get—and use—contraceptives (birth control) when you start having sex.

Healing after a cesarean birth

If you have a c-section, most of the things listed above will apply to you. But there are a few more things to know.

- **You will hurt for a while.** It takes 4 to 6 weeks for the cut to heal. You will have a checkup 6 weeks afterward.

- **Take care of your incision (cut).** Ask the doctor or nurse how to keep it clean and when you can get it wet. Be gentle with it, no scrubbing or clothes that rub against it. Watch for signs of infection—if it feels hot, turns bright red, oozes, or opens up, you need to call your doctor.

- **Get lots of rest.** It takes longer to heal if you get overtired. Rest as much as you can. Use your energy to feed and cuddle your baby.

- **Don't lift** anything heavier than your baby for the first few weeks. Keep the things you need within easy reach.

- **Find ways of holding baby** that are don't press on the cut. Put a pillow on your belly when holding him in your lap. Or try the football hold—baby's body goes under your arm and his feet are behind you.

- **Get some gentle exercise every day.** Deep breathing, stretching, and walking are enough at first. Talk to your doctor or midwife about what is safe.

- **To lessen pain when you sit up,** stand up, sit down, or bend over, press a firm pillow over your stitches. Press your hand (or the pillow) over the incision when you

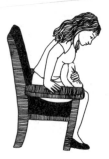

Hold a pillow over your stitches when you get up. This will make it less painful to get up.

laugh, cough, sneeze, or move suddenly. It will help limit the pain.

◆ **Ask your doctor or midwife** when it is safe to use stairs, exercise more, or drive. Accept all offers to help around the house with cooking, cleaning, and the laundry.

Breast care

Your breasts will keep changing after you have your baby. Wear a bra or top with good support when you feel like you need it. Other times, you may be more comfortable in something soft or loose. Wear what feels good, especially if your breasts are sore. See Chapter 12 for tips on breast care while breastfeeding, formula feeding, or both.

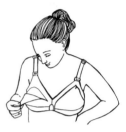

A bra with good support

Keep up your healthy habits

Follow the healthy food habits you started in pregnancy (Chapter 4). You need to eat well to get back your strength and energy. Eat plenty of protein and calcium from meat, fish, beans, tofu, nuts, seeds, milk, and cheese. If you are breastfeeding twins or triplets, you will need to eat more to make larger amounts of breast milk.

Start exercising gently

Protect your back. Keep a straight back and bend your knees when lifting your baby. Try to stand up straight when you carry him. Make sure the baby carrier you use has good back support for you and fits baby well, too. Other exercises will help, too, like those shown in the pictures.

Walking is the best way to start getting back in shape. You can wear your baby in a carrier. He'll like the ride and the gentle movement. If you had a c-section, ask your doctor before starting to exercise.

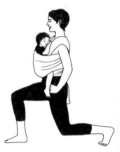

You could take baby with you to an exercise class for new moms.

Continue to avoid alcohol and other drugs

Being a parent can be hard, but using alcohol, cigarettes, and other drugs doesn't make it easier. They can make it harder for you to handle the tough parts of parenting.

If you are breastfeeding, these drugs can hurt your baby's brain and growth. Breast milk carries alcohol, nicotine, and other drugs to your baby.

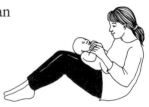

Sit with baby on your thighs, then lean back slowly with a straight back.

Smoke in the air can give him baby problems, too. Babies of smokers have more colds, ear infections, and a higher risk of SIDS. Anyone who smokes should do so outside the house and not in the car with baby.

E-cigarettes may not be much healthier than regular cigarettes. Little is known about the vapor that goes into the air. The liquid inside or in refills is very poisonous to kids who might touch it or drink it.

Your own six-week checkup

Your baby's first checkups are very important, but so is your own 6-week checkup! Your doctor or midwife will want to see you about six weeks after your baby was born. He will want to check how your body is healing and how you are feeling. This is a good time to talk about breastfeeding, exercise, sex, and birth control. So make an appointment now. If you have questions sooner, don't wait until this visit to ask them. It's okay to call at any time.

It is also important for you to go in for a checkup one year after birth. This will help make sure your body has gotten back on track after baby.

Sex after baby

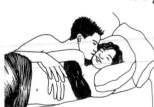

Every woman is different when it comes to having sex after baby. It is a good idea to wait at least four to six weeks before having sex or putting anything in your vagina. This gives your body time to heal inside.

It's important to wait until you feel ready. Some women are ready for sex after just a few weeks. Other women feel that they should wait a few months or more. Sex may feel different than before. Talk to your partner and take things slowly. There are other ways to be close.

Some things that could affect your feelings about having sex soon after you give birth are:

- Your body and feelings are very tired from taking care of your baby.
- Sex can seem scary when your body (vagina, bottom, or c-section cut) is sore or healing.
- Your breasts may leak milk or be sore.

Call your doctor or midwife if you want to have sex before your six-week checkup. He can help you make sure your body is ready. He can also help you choose some kind of birth control, even if you haven't had your period yet.

Remember, the right time for sex is when you feel ready and want to. If some time has passed and you still don't want it, it could be a sign of depression. See page 251 to learn more.

Don't wait to think about birth control

The best time to think about birth control is before you start having sex again. Many women think they don't need it right away and end up pregnant again too soon.

Do some family planning. This means you and your partner should talk about if and when you want another baby. If you do want more kids, it's best to wait until your baby is at least 18 months old before you get pregnant again. This gives your body time to heal and get strong again after birth. It helps your next baby be healthier. And your first child will be over age 2 and better able to cope with a new sister or brother.

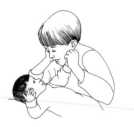

"Our first child was almost 4 when our second was born. He really enjoyed having a new baby brother."

Facts about family planning

Decide what kind of birth control to use to make sure you don't get pregnant before you are ready. However, there are a number of ways people try to keep from getting pregnant that you can't count on:

- Breastfeeding
- Withdrawal of the man's penis before he comes
- Thinking you can't get pregnant until after your menstrual periods start again
- The rhythm method can only work after your periods are completely regular again. This probably won't work all the time.

There are many methods that work very well. Find out more from your provider or go to Planned Parenthood. Choose one that fits your lifestyle and your long-term family plans.

If you start having sex before you see your doctor, use condoms and spermicide* (foam or jelly) together, or a spermicidal sponge. They cost very little and can be bought at

*Spermicide: Medication that kills the male sperm.

drug stores without a prescription. These are not as effective as other methods for long-term use.

A condom is the only kind of birth control that also can prevent sexually-transmitted diseases. There are condoms for women as well as for men.

Emergency contraception

If you have unprotected sex (or if a condom breaks), there are two birth control options to keep you from getting pregnant. They must be used within five days of having sex. They are only for emergencies, not for regular birth control.

The emergency pill ("morning-after pill") works best the sooner you take it. Women age 17 and older can buy it at some pharmacies without a prescription. A copper IUD may also be put into your uterus as emergency birth control. Call your doctor, nurse, or midwife if you need emergency contraception.

How are you feeling?

Having a new baby changes your life in many ways. It is a very emotional time with highs and lows. For some people it is a happy time but for others it can be very hard. There are so many new things to learn and your baby needs you all the time. It is okay to have mixed feelings.

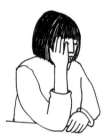

Get help if you start to feel depressed.

Many parents feel upset or sad after their child is born. They may cry easily, get mad over little things, or have trouble eating and sleeping in the first few weeks. This is called the "baby blues" and 8 out of 10 parents go through it. But, if these feelings last longer, get worse, or make it hard for you to care for yourself or your baby, it may be something more serious.

Mood disorders* in pregnancy or after giving birth

*Mood disorder:
Emotional illness or condition.

*Postpartum:
The time after a baby's birth.

Mood disorders happen to many parents during pregnancy or after baby is born. Postpartum* depression and anxiety are the most common, but there are others, too. For some people, this is the first time they have had these problems.

Watch each other for any of the warning signs above. Get help as soon as you feel your mood changing. Try not to hide from it or be a superhero. It's important not to wait.

Warning Signs: Is It More Than Just Baby Blues?

Please check the things you or your partner feels often, even if they don't feel serious to you. Some may be hard to admit. Be honest with yourself.
Have you had a mood disorder (like depression or anxiety) before?

- ☐ Do you feel very sad?
- ☐ Do you feel mad at the people around you over little things?
- ☐ Is it hard for you to feel close to your baby?
- ☐ Do you feel panic or are you always worried about how you are caring for baby?
- ☐ Is it hard for you to eat or sleep?
- ☐ Do you feel very happy one minute and very upset the next?
- ☐ Do you have bad thoughts in your mind that you can't get rid of?
- ☐ Do you feel like you're "going crazy"?
- ☐ Do you feel like you can't be a good parent?
- ☐ Are you afraid you might hurt yourself or your baby?

If the answer is yes to any one of these, tell your provider. You may have a mood disorder. It can happen to anyone, including dads or partners, and is very common. There is help! You don't need to suffer.

It can be hard to admit to or talk about these feelings. It can even be hard to believe that you have a problem. Many people try to just "live with it" or pretend they are okay. Some people need others to get help for them because they are too upset to call for themselves. Remember, this can happen to moms or partners and is hard on the whole family.

How does a mood disorder happen?

It can happen from too much stress, too little sleep, bad eating habits, money trouble, or family problems. It is more likely if you have had a birth that was very hard, scary, or not what you wanted. However, a mood disorder is more common if you or a relative has had depression, anxiety, bipolar, or obsessive-compulsive disorder in the past. It is also more likely if you have been abused, even as a child.

"After my first baby was born, I spent a whole year being really worried that I wasn't doing everything right. It was awful. With my new baby, I got some medicine for my anxiety. What a difference! I feel like I'm a much better mom now."

What to do if you're having a hard time

Call **1-800-944-4773** to get support from Postpartum International.

If you are in crisis and need help right away, call the National Suicide Prevention Hotline at **1-800-273-8255**. In an emergency, call 9-1-1.

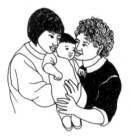

Tell your provider if either you or your partner has any of the signs above. Tell her you want to talk to someone who works with mood disorders. The sooner you get professional help, the better for you and your baby. There is no need to suffer.

Ways to help yourself

Take care of yourself. Try to eat well and get some sleep each day (at least four or five hours of non-stop sleep in a row). Get up, move around, and get out of the house. Fresh air and exercise can help with stress.

Remember—this is not your fault. You didn't make this happen. You're not alone. It will get better.

Be around people you like. Just because you love someone doesn't mean he or she is good at helping you feel relaxed. Ask people to visit who make you laugh, whom you trust, and who will support you. Share your feelings, good or bad, with them. Put off stressful visits until you or your partner feels better.

Have a plan for support. Say "yes" when people offer to help. Think of things people can do for you and ask them. It could be something big like helping to pay your bills or something small like bringing a meal or walking your dog.

Talk to others who have gone through this. It helps to know you're not alone. Ask around in your group of friends. Also find a support group in your area or online.

No one is a perfect parent!

Are you or your partner worried about doing things wrong? You do not have to know all the answers. You will learn as you go along. You do not have to do it alone.

You can get advice from friends, relatives, neighbors, your health clinic, and many organizations. There are parent groups, lactation consultants, and playgroups to turn to. There is a lot of information that you can trust in books, videos, and Internet sites.

Just remember, you are the parents and get to decide which advice is best for your family.

If Your Partner Seems Depressed

What to say to your partner that can help:

- *You're not alone. I'm here for you.*
- *You will get better. We'll get through this.*
- *This isn't your fault.*
- *I love you so much. The baby loves you so much.*
- *I'm sorry you're hurting.*
- *You're a great parent. I love how you stroke baby's head while he's nursing.*
- *As your partner gets better, tell him or her the ways you see them getting better.*

Things people say that are *not* helpful:

- *Snap out of it.*
- *Try feeling happy.*
- *Just calm down.*
- *Think about all you have to be thankful for.*

Tips for partners

This is a big time for you. You are playing a huge role in making sure mom and baby are taken care of. You also need to make sure that you take care of yourself! Both of you will need to have patience and get rest when you can. There are two big things to pay attention to: sex and depression.

Talking about sex

It can be hard to talk about sex after baby. First, read page 248. This can be a very hard issue for moms. Some women find that all of their emotions are about caring for the new baby. Others may really want to have sex but their bodies may not be ready. It is very important for you to be patient and kind. It's okay to tell her that you want to be close again, but don't push her. Find other ways of being close for a while.

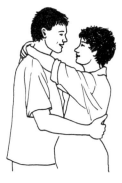

When you do have sex, be sure to use protection. It's important not to get pregnant again too soon.

More tips for partners:

- ◆ Read this chapter to learn what mom is going through after birth. It will help you understand and know how to help.
- ◆ Put phone numbers for her provider, baby's doctor, and a lactation consultant in your phone or on the door of the fridge. Offer to call if either of you is worried.
- ◆ Find a local group for dads or partners with babies for play or support.

Affirmations for parents to remember

I am learning more every day about being good to myself.

I have friends I can call on when I need support or someone to talk with.

I am being the best parent I can be, knowing what I know now.

Nobody is perfect. My child will forgive any small mistakes I make.

I enjoy seeing how my baby learns and grows from week to week.

I'm not the first person who has been depressed during this time. I can ask for help.

My baby gives me the chance to become a new person.

I am a good parent.

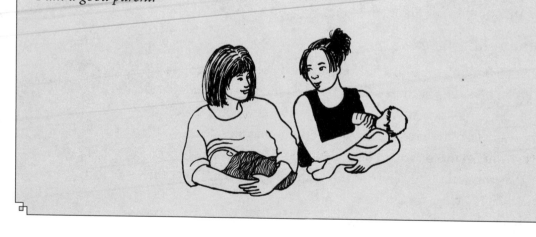

Chapter 17

Resources to Help You

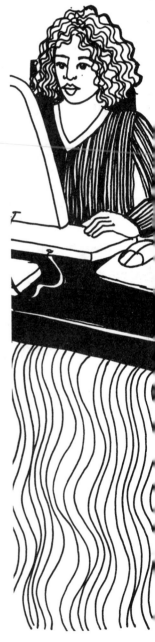

When you need to know more

Your health care provider is your best source of information. But there's a lot you can learn on your own. There's much more to know about pregnancy, birth, and baby care than fits into this book. This chapter gives you lots more ways to learn more.

You may hear or read things that seem very different from what you have read here or heard from your health care provider. Be sure to check it out. Ask your health care provider before making big changes in what you do. Ask questions and use your common sense.

Look in this chapter for:

Help where you live, page 256

Websites and national resources, page 257

Women's health resources, page 257

    Childbirth—Birth classes

    Mood disorders, Crisis hotlines

    Family planning

    LGBTQ families, Teens

    Twins, Multiples

Baby-care resources, page 259

    Breastfeeding

    Crying

    Safety: in car, when sleeping

    Vaccines

Books to keep handy, page 261

Glossary: Words to know, page 263

Getting Help

You may already know about some of the organizations listed here. They all have useful services for pregnant women and new parents. They can help you find other resources. Many can be found on the Internet (see National Resources list).

Some of the best help will come from organizations or agencies in your own city or town. Many national groups have local chapters. Their phone numbers and addresses can be found in your phone book. Look under "Health," "Education," or "Government" listings.

You also can find local links on national organization websites. Your health care provider, public health department, or hospital social worker will also be able to help.

Resources where you live

Breastfeeding: Lactation consultants, La Leche League groups

Childbirth education classes: ICEA, Lamaze, your hospital

Churchs, synagogues, or other places of worship: Parent support programs

Community health centers: Prenatal and well-baby care

Community colleges: Parent education

Community information lines: Referral to local services

Crisis hotlines: Telephone help and information service for people who are very upset, sad, or angry, including abused women.

Family planning: Public health clinics, Planned Parenthood clinics

Hospitals: Classes for childbirth, baby care, and infant first aid, social workers

Mental health center: Counseling and support groups for people with problems

Parent support groups: Groups set up by different organizations where parents support and help one another; some for new parents and others for parents of children with specific disabilities

Public health department: Clinics, prenatal care, well-baby care, parent education, home visits

Public library: Books, pamphlets, DVDs, CDs, and lists of educational programs on prenatal and family health

Safe Kids Coalition: Car seat and other child safety information and programs

School nurse: Help for students having health issues

WIC (Special Supplemental Nutrition Program for Women, Infants, and Children): Nutrition program for pregnant or nursing women and their young children

Your health plan: May include a nurse hotline or health information service

Websites and national resources

You can learn a lot from the Internet. But, be careful where you look. Find websites you can trust. Major health or government organizations are good sources. All of the websites listed here have information you can trust. These pages may have links to other helpful websites, too. Many sites also have Spanish pages.

If you do not have a computer, try your local library or community center. They probably will have computers you can use and people who can help you find what you need.

WARNING: Be careful using the web. Look for how new the information is and who wrote it. Check out the sponsors of the site. Some sites may look official but do not give correct information. Some mainly sell things or give you only one side of an issue. Many pages are out of date. When in doubt, ask your provider about information you find.

Web addresses often change. If any sites listed here do not show you what you are looking for, do a search for the name of the agency or the topic you want to find (such as "childbirth").

Women—Pregnant and new moms' health resources

Childbirth—Birth classes

ICEA (International Childbirth Education Association): Classes in childbirth preparation and parenting. Find childbirth teachers, *www.icea.org*

Lamaze International: Find local teachers of classes in this method of natural childbirth; *www.lamaze.org*; 1-800-368-4404

Childbirth—Doula care

Dona International: About doulas and finding trained doulas, *www.dona.org*; 1-888-788-DONA (1-888-788-3662)

Depression and mood disorders

National Women's Health Resource Center: Search for depression, *www.healthywomen.org*; 1-877-986-9472

Postpartum Support International: 1-800-944-4773; *www.postpartum.net* Español: *www.postpartum.net/En-Español.aspx*

Baby Blues Connection: 1-800-5578375; *www.babybluesconnection.org*

One website covers it all

One reliable place to find information on most health and safety topics is through the National Institute of Health at: *www.medlineplus.gov.* It also has a large section in Spanish.

Crisis center hotlines

In an emergency, you can call 9-1-1 for help.

National Suicide Prevention Hotline: 1-800-273-8255

National Safe Haven Alliance Hotline: Help for women who need to give up their baby. 1-888-510-2229; *www.nationalsafehavenalliance.org*

Women'sLaw.org: state-by-state legal information and resources for abused women, *www.womenslaw.org*

National Domestic Violence Hotline, 1-800-799-SAFE (1-800-799-7233), (English and Spanish); *www.thehotline.com.org*

National Child Abuse Hotline: 1-800-4-A-CHILD (1-800-422-4453)

National Fussy Baby Warmline: 1-888-431-BABY (1-888-431-2229)

Family planning

National Family Planning & Reproductive Health Assn.: Find a clinic near you; *www.nationalfamilyplanning.org*

Not Too Late—Emergency contraception: *www.NOT-2-LATE.com*

Planned Parenthood Federation of America: birth control, family planning, and women's health: *www.plannedparenthood.org*; 1-800-230-PLAN (1-800-230-7526); English and Spanish.

Health insurance

Affordable Care Act, includes how to apply for Medicaid or Children's Health Insurance Program (CHIP), *www.healthcare.gov*

Health plans from insurance companies, *www.insurance.healthplans.com*; 1-800-372-1458

LGBTQ families

LGBT Families: *www.lgbtfamilies.info*

Human Rights Campaign: *www.hrc.org/topics/parenting*

Nutrition, food safety

US Dept. of Agriculture (USDA): *www.choosemyplate.gov/pregnancy-breastfeeding.html*

WIC: www.fns.usda.gov/wic/ (click on "How to Apply" to find state contacts and toll-free numbers)

Mercury in fish: www.water.epa.gov/scitech/swguidance/fishshellfish/fishadvisories/index.cfm

Parenting support

Nurse-Family Partnership: Helping first-time parents succeed. Services in some cities in almost all states, *www.nursefamilypartnership.org*

Parents as Teachers: Supporting new moms and their partners to strengthen parenting skills. In communities in all states; *www.parentsasteachers.org*

Child and Family Web Guide, Tufts Univ.: *www.cfw.tufts.edu* (go to Parenting)

Pregnancy and Childbirth

American College of Nurse-Midwives: *www.midwife.org/For-Women-Splash*

Evidence Based Birth:
www.evidencebasedbirth.com

March of Dimes: *www.marchofdimes.com*

Office on Women's Health:
www.womenshealth.gov

Lamaze: *www.lamaze.org/*

National Women's Health Resource
Center: *www.healthywomen.org*;
1-877-986-9472

Maternity Center Association: Clear
discussions of current issues, like
non-emergency cesarean delivery,
based on current research:
1-212-777-5000;
www.maternitywise.org

Quitting alcohol, drug, tobacco use

Drug and Substance Abuse Treatment:
www.samhsa.gov; Hotline
1-800-662-HELP (1-800-662-4357)

Baby-Care Resources

American Academy of Pediatrics (AAP):
www.healthychildren.org

American Academy of Pediatrics:
www.healthychildren.org

American Academy of Family
Physicians: *www.familydoctor.org*

KidsHealth (Nemours):
www.kidshealth.org (also in Spanish)

Babywearing

Babywearing International:
www.babywearinginternational.org

Birth defects and disability

March of Dimes, News Moms Need,
www.newsmomsneed.marchofdimes.org

Quitting smoking (CDC): *www.cdc.gov/
tobacco/campaign/tips/quit-smoking*;
1-800-784-8669;
Spanish: 1-855-335-3569

National Council on Alcoholism and
Drug Dependence: *www.ncadd.org/*;
1-800-622-2255

Teen parents—See Parenting support

National Women's Law Center: (Go to
Our Issues, Education & Title IX,
Pregnant & Parenting Students)
www.nwlc.org

Twins, Multiples

Mothers of Twins Clubs:
www.nomotc.org

Working while pregnant and mothering

Babygate: your rights in the workplace:
www.babygate.abetterbalance.org

Breastfeeding

La Leche League: Learn about
breastfeeding, or find help near you:
www.lalecheleague.org;
1-800-LALECHE (1-800-525-3243)

Breastfeeding USA: *breastfeedingusa.org*

KellyMom: *www.kellymom.com*

National Women's Health Resource
Center: *www.healthywomen.org*;
1-877-986-9472

AAP: *www.healthychildren.org* (search
for breastfeeding)

Human Milk Banking Association of
North America: *www.hmbana.org*

Human Milk 4 Human Babies:
www.hm4hb.net

Eats on Feets: *www.eatsonfeets.org*

Car seats—See Safety in the car

Child abuse

National Child Abuse Hotline:
1-800-4-A-CHILD (1-800-422-4453)

Babies' development

Zero to Three:
www.zerotothree.org/child-development

CDC Child Development site,
*www.cdc.gov/ncbddd/childdevelopment
/index.html*

Make the First Five Years Count:
www.easterseals.com/mtffc

Crying

Period of Purple Crying:
www.purplecrying.info

The Fussy Baby Network
www.erikson.edu/fussybaby/;
1-888-431-BABY (1-888-431-2229)

Immunizations—See Vaccines

Poisoning

Call 9-1-1 if child won't wake up or is
not breathing

National Poison Center: 1-800-222-1222

American Assn. of Poison Control
Centers, *www.aaapcc.org/children.htm*

Safety—General

Safe Kids Worldwide: Learn to prevent
injuries or find a local program: *www.
safekids.org*; 202-662-0600

Make Safe Happen:
www.makesafehappen.com

Safety in the car

AAP: *www.healthychildren.org* (go to
Safety & Prevention, On-the-Go)
Also in Spanish

SeatCheck.org: Find a car seat check
near you. *www.seatcheck.org*;
1-866-SEAT-CHECK
(1-866-732-8243) Also in Spanish

National Highway Traffic Safety
Administration:1-800-424-9393;
www.safercar.gov/parents/

The Car Seat Lady:
www.thecarseatlady.com

Kids and Cars:
www.kidsandcars.org

SafetyBeltSafe U.S.A.: Helpline:
1-800-745-SAFE (1-800-745-7233);
Helpline-Spanish:1-800-745-SANO
(1-800-745-7266); *www.carseat.org*

Automotive Safety Program: car safety
information for infants and children
with special needs;
*www.preventinjury.org/Special-Needs
-Transportation*

Safety at home

Safe Kids Worldwide:
www.safekids.org

Consumer Product Safety Commission:
www.saferproducts.gov;
1-800-638-2772

KidsHealth (Nemours):
www.kidshealth.org; Also in Spanish

Baby proof home: *www.parents.com*
(search for baby proofing)

Safe sleep

Safe to Sleep Campaign;
   www.nichd.nih.gov/sts/

CDC Sudden Unexpected Infant Death:
   www.cdc.gov/sids/parents-caregivers
   .htm

Co-sleeping: Mother-Baby Behavioral
   Sleep Laboratory, Univ. of Notre Dame:
   www.cosleeping.nd.edu/

Twins and Multiples

Mothers of Twins:
   www.motheroftwins.com

Multiples of America: *www.nomotc.org*

BabyCenter: *www.babycenter.com*

Vaccines

CDC Vaccines and Immunizations:
   www.cdc.gov/vaccines/parents/

Other sites with good advice

Babycenter.com and *Parenting.com*:
   These are not expert resources, but
   have some good information. Ask
   your provider about things you learn
   from them.

Using social media

"There's an app for that!"

Many health programs are making "apps" to use on cell phones and tablets. You can get weekly updates on how your baby is growing, time contractions, learn CPR, or even find car seat tips this way.

These programs can be fun and even come in handy. Check them out with the same care as other resources. And, don't let them replace talking to your healthcare provider, especially about health or safety issues.

Books to keep handy

This book gives the **basics** every woman needs to know during pregnancy and the first months after birth. There are many books that have more details. Here are a few books that we think you would find useful. Find them in your local library or bookstore.

Look for the newest version of a book. This will help make sure you get the best information. Some books about pregnancy, general baby care, behavior, or development are classic. They do not really go out of date. We include these because we hope every pregnant woman or new parent will get wisdom from them. Often you can find these in libraries.

You may want to have one "fat book" of information on all the topics that you might need someday, like ear aches or sore throats. In bookstores, you will find a huge number of books about pregnancy and baby care. We list a few below that we think are special in some way.

Tips for choosing reliable health books:

◆ Look for text that's easy for you to read and pictures that help you learn

◆ Find an edition that's been published in about the last five years, except classics. (The copyright date is on the back of the title page.)

- Avoid old editions: they may be cheaper but will not give the best advice.

Open a book and read a few pages before buying it. Compare a few books. Check what they say about certain things like avoiding c-sections or keeping kids rear-facing in car seats until age 2. Some books will be easier or more fun to read than others.

Remember, you may find advice that confuses you. Be sure to ask your provider about it.

General References (fat books)

These books cover all aspects of medical topics without being overwhelming. They are trustworthy, fairly easy to read, and have plenty of helpful pictures. These would be good to have on your shelf.

Your Pregnancy and Childbirth—Month to Month, American College of Obstetrics and Gynecology, 2010

Pregnancy, Childbirth and the Newborn, Penny Simkin, PT, April Bolding, and Ann Keppler, RN, MN, and others 2010 (2015 edition coming soon)

The Healthy Pregnancy Book, William Sears and Martha Sears, 2013

Caring for Your Baby and Young Child, Birth to Age 5, American Academy of Pediatrics, Steven Shelov and Tanya Altmann, 2009

Prenatal Care books

A Child is Born, Lennart Nilsson, 2004

Complete Book of Pregnancy and Childbirth, Sheila Kitzinger, 2003

Our Bodies, Ourselves: Pregnancy and Birth, Boston Women's Health Book Collective. 2008

When You're Expecting Twins, Triplets, or Quads, Dr. Barbara Luke & Tamara Eberlein, 2010

Ask a Midwife, Catherine Parker-Littler, 2008

The Simple Guide to Having a Baby: A Step-by-Step Illustrated Guide to Having a Baby, Janet Whalley and Penny Simkin, 2012

The Birth Partner, Penny Simkin, 2008

Especially For Teens

Your Pregnancy & Newborn Journey: A Guide for Pregnant Teens, Jeanne Lindsay and Jean Brunelli

Nurturing Your Newborn: Young Parents' Guide to Baby's First Month, Jeanne Lindsay and Jean Brunelli

Teen Dads: Rights, Responsibilities & Joys, Jeanne Lindsay and Jean Brunelli

Your Baby's First Year, A Guide for Teenage Parents, Jeanne Lindsay and Jean Brunelli

My Pregnant Girlfriend, Charles Ordoqui, 2012

Baby Care books

Heading Home with Your Newborn, Laura A. Jana, MD, and Jennifer Shu, MD, 2010, American Academy of Pediatrics

Baby 411: Clear Answers & Smart Advice for Your Baby's First Year, Ari Brown and Denise Fields, 2013

Premature Baby Book, William Sears, MD and others, 2010

The Multiples Manual, Lynn Lorenz, 2007

The Magic Years, Selma Fraiberg, 2008

Touchpoints: Birth to 3: Your Child's Emotional and Behavioral Development, T. Berry Brazelton, MD, 2006

Year After Childbirth: Surviving and Enjoying the First Year of Motherhood, Sheila Kitzinger, 1994

Breastfeeding books

The Womanly Art of Breastfeeding, La Leche League International, 2010

Breastfeeding made Simple; Seven Natural Laws for Nursing Mothers, Nancy Mohrbacher and Kathleen Kendal-Tackett, 2010

Nursing Mother, Working Mother, Gale Pryor and Kathleen Huggins, 2007

Glossary: words to know

Abdomen – The part of your body below your ribs and above your legs. Contains your stomach, uterus, and other organs.

Abortion – Ending of a pregnancy, which may be natural (miscarriage) or done by a doctor (induced).

AIDS – Acquired Immunodeficiency Syndrome, a fatal disease passed from person to person most often by having sex or sharing needles. May be passed to an unborn baby.

Air Bag – A safety device for front seat car passengers that is hidden in the dashboard and opens if a crash occurs.

Amniocentesis – A test of the fluid inside the bag of waters, showing certain things about your unborn baby's health.

Amniotic fluid – Liquid in the amniotic sac.

Amniotic sac – The "bag of waters" inside the uterus, in which the baby grows.

Anesthesia – Various drugs used to reduce or eliminate pain.

Antibodies – Cells made in a person's body to fight disease. A baby's first antibodies come from mother's colostrum and milk.

Aspirin – A non-prescription drug that lessens pain and lowers fever.

Areola – The dark area around the nipple.

Bag of waters – The amniotic sac in which your baby grows inside the uterus.

Birth canal – Your vagina, the opening through which your baby will be born.

Birth control – Ways to keep from getting pregnant when you have sex. Examples: condom, diaphragm, pills, IUD.

Birth defect – Baby's health problem that happens before birth or during birth. May have lasting effects.

Blood pressure – The force of blood pumped by the heart through a person's blood vessels. High blood pressure means the heart is pumping extra hard.

Bloody show – A small amount of mucus and blood (the "mucus plug") that comes from your cervix before labor begins.

Braxton-Hicks contractions – Tightening and relaxing of the muscle of your uterus during the last few months of pregnancy.

Breech birth – Birth of a baby who is not head-down. (Often buttocks first.)

Calcium – A mineral in foods needed to make bones and teeth grow strong.

Calories – Energy in foods. Some kinds of foods have more calories than others.

Car seat – A seat specially designed and tested for use to protect infants or children from injury in a vehicle crash.

Certified Nurse-midwife – A nurse who delivers babies, who has been specially trained as a midwife and passed a national test.

Cervix – The neck (opening) of the uterus (womb). Your baby is pushed out through the cervix into the vagina during delivery.

Cesarean section – Delivery of a baby by making a cut through the woman's belly into the uterus. Short name is c-section.

Child safety seat (child restraint) – See "car seat."

Circumcision – Surgery to take off the loose skin around the top of a baby boy's penis.

Colostrum – The thin, yellowish liquid that comes out of a woman's nipples during late pregnancy and the first few days after birth.

Conception – The beginning of a baby's growth, when the mother's egg unites with the father's sperm.

Condom – A rubber or latex tube with a closed end that is used during sex to prevent pregnancy and diseases that can be passed during sex. A male condom is put on the penis just before sex. A female condom is put into the vagina or anus just before sex.

Constipation – When bowel movements are very hard and do not come regularly.

Contraception – See Birth control.

Contractions – The tightening of the muscle of your uterus.

Core – The main part of your body (chest, shoulders, abdomen, back).

C-section – See Cesarean section.

Development – The ways in which the baby's mind learns and the body grows and changes.

Diarrhea – Bowel movements that are very soft and watery and come more often than usual.

Digestion – The changing of your food in your mouth, stomach, and intestines for use by your body.

Dilation – The stretching open of the cervix during the first stage of labor.

Discharge – Liquid that comes out of your body, like blood or mucus from your vagina.

Doula – A person trained to help parents during and after delivery.

Drop – The sinking of the unborn baby down into the pelvis before birth begins.

Drugs – Many kinds of things that affect your body or feelings, such as medicines, or substances like alcohol, tobacco, or illegal (street) drugs.

Due date – The date when a baby is expected to be born.

Effacement – The thinning of the cervix during the first stage of labor.

Embryo – Word used for a tiny unborn baby during the first eight weeks of its growth.

Engagement – The sinking (dropping) of the uterus down into the pelvis before birth.

Engorgement – Hard and painful breasts when they are starting to produce milk.

Episiotomy – A cut made in the skin around the vagina to widen the opening and help the baby to be born.

Family physician or practitioner – A doctor who takes care of the health of people of all ages.

Family planning – Using a birth control method to control the number of children in the family, and getting pregnant when a person or couple chooses.

Fertility – The ability to conceive a child.

Fetal monitor – A machine that tells how the unborn baby's heart is beating, used to check the baby's health inside the uterus.

Fetus – Word used for the unborn baby, from 8 weeks to birth at about 40 weeks.

Fiber – A part of food that helps bowel movements be soft and regular.

Fontanelles – Soft spots in the skull of a newborn baby. They close slowly over many months.

Formula – Special milk for bottle-feeding. Made to be much like breast milk.

Genetic counseling – Help for people with health problems that may be passed down to their children.

Genetic defects – Health problems that are passed down from parent to child to grandchild through genetic matter in the cells.

Genitals – A boy's penis and girl's vulva.

Gestational Diabetes – A type of diabetes that happens in pregnancy and can cause problems for mother and baby if not managed.

Group B Streptococcus (GBS) – A type of bacteria ("Strep") that can live in the vagina and can seriously harm a newborn baby.

Health care provider – A person trained to take care of people's health and illness (nurses, doctors, midwives).

Heartburn – A burning feeling in your chest caused by acid from your stomach going up into the esophagus (tube from mouth to stomach).

Hemorrhoids – Veins at your anus (opening where stool comes out) that get swollen and feel itchy or painful.

Hormones – Substances made by organs in the body that control how it works and feels.

Immune system – The body system that fights disease by making antibodies.

Immunization (vaccination, shot) – Delivery of a vaccine that helps the body make antibodies to fight against a disease.

Incubator – A special bed for a baby who needs extra care.

Induce, induction – Start contractions with drugs or other means.

Infection – A sore or illness caused by germs that harm your body.

Intact penis – a penis that hasn't been circumcised.

Iron – A mineral in foods that helps your blood carry oxygen to your baby's body.

Isolette – See Incubator.

Isopropyl alcohol – The kind of alcohol used to kill germs (not safe to drink).

Kangaroo care – Cuddling a baby against the parent's bare chest so they are skin-to-skin. Especially good for preemies.

Kegel – An exercise for the muscles of your perineum, around the vaginal opening.

Labor – The work your uterus does to open the cervix and push the baby down into the birth canal.

LATCH system – Lower Anchors and Tethers for Children; a way of installing a car seat in a vehicle using special connectors on the car seat and anchors in the vehicle.

Lactation specialist – A person with special training and knowledge about breastfeeding (lactation).

Lanugo – Soft, short hair growing on the body of a fetus and newborn baby.

Medication – Drugs (medicines) that a doctor prescribes for you or that you can buy at a drug store.

Menstrual period – The bloody lining of the uterus that flows from a woman's vagina every month.

Midwife – A person who helps women have their babies. (Not a doctor.)

Miscarriage (spontaneous abortion) – When an embryo or fetus is born too young to survive (before 20 weeks.)

Mood disorder – An emotional illness or condition that can affect everyday life.

Morning sickness – Name for the feeling of nausea, often with vomiting, in the first few months of pregnancy.

Mucus plug – The thick blob of mucus that fills the cervix during pregnancy.

Multiple pregnancy – Twins, triplets, or more babies born at the same time.

Neonatal Intensive Care Unit (NICU) – The hospital nursery for preemies or those with serious medical problems.

Non-aspirin pain reliever – Acetaminophen, a drug better than aspirin for children with pain or fever; "Tylenol" is one common brand.

Nurse-midwife – A nurse with special training to deliver babies.

Nurse practitioner – A nurse with special training to do some aspects of health care, working with a doctor.

Nursing – Another word for breastfeeding.

Nutrients – Things in foods that keep you healthy.

Obstetrician-Gynecologist – A doctor who takes care of women's health. An obstetrician specializes in prenatal care and delivery of babies. A gynecologist specializes in the health of women's uterus and sex organs.

Pediatrician – A doctor who takes care of children's health.

Pelvic exam – A way for your doctor or nurse midwife to check your vagina and uterus by pressing on your belly and reaching up inside your vagina, and by looking inside.

Pelvis – Your hip bones inside which your uterus sits. Your vagina (birth canal) goes through a wide opening in these bones.

Perinatal – The time before and after a baby's birth.

Perineum – The skin and muscles around the opening of the vagina. Also called the pelvic floor.

Period – A short word for menstrual period.

Postpartum: The time after a baby's birth.

Placenta – The organ that connects the mother's body with her fetus, moving food and oxygen from the mother's blood to the unborn baby's blood.

Preemie – A short term for a preterm infant.

Pregnancy – The nine months when a woman has a baby growing inside her uterus.

Pregnancy-induced hypertension (PIH) – High blood pressure during pregnancy. May lead to preeclampsia if not treated.

Prenatal – During pregnancy (when a baby is inside the mother).

Prescription – An order for medicine from your doctor.

Preterm (premature) – A baby born early, before the 37th week of pregnancy.

Protein – Substances in food that make your body grow well and work properly.

Reflexes – Movements of the body that happen automatically.

Reflux – Acid from the stomach that backs up into the esophagus (tube from the mouth to the stomach).

Sexually-transmitted disease (STD) – A disease passed from one person to another when they have sex.

Spinal cord – The main nerve in the body that goes up the middle of the spine or backbone. It connects the brain to the rest of the body.

Stillbirth – When a baby dies before or during birth (after 20 weeks).

Stool – A bowel movement.

Sudden infant death syndrome (SIDS) – Death of a sleeping baby when all other causes have been ruled out.

Support system – The people in your life who help you in times of need.

Swaddling – Wrapping a newborn baby snugly in a thin blanket for comfort.

Symptoms – Changes in your body or how you feel (like pain, itching, or bleeding). These help your provider know what health problem you have.

Temporal artery thermometer: A thermometer that senses temperature from the artery under the forehead skin.

Trimester – A three-month period. A full pregnancy has three trimesters.

Tympanic thermometer: A thermometer that senses temperature from the ear opening.

Ultrasound – Special tool used to see inside your body to find out how your unborn baby is doing or growing.

Umbilical cord – The long tube that attaches the placenta to the unborn baby's body at the navel (belly button). It carries food and oxygen from the mother's body and wastes from the baby's body.

Uterus – The womb, the organ in which an unborn baby grows.

Vaccine – Substance given to immunize against disease. (See immunizations.)

Vagina – The opening in a woman's body where menstrual flow comes out and a man puts his penis during sex. Also, the birth canal through which a baby is born.

Vaginal birth – The natural type of birth, in which the baby passes through the cervix and vagina.

Varicose veins – Blue, swollen veins that itch or ache, that often occur in the legs during pregnancy.

VBAC – Vaginal Birth After a Cesarean.

Vernix – Grayish-white, cheese-like cream covering the skin of a newborn baby.

Vomiting – Throwing up stomach contents.

Vulva – The female genitals around the opening of the vagina.

Well-baby, Well-child checkup – Regular health visits for babies and children who are not ill. Checkups cover health, development, immunizations, and screening tests.

WIC (Women, Infants, and Children) Program – A federal nutrition program that provides food and educational support for eligible women and children up to age 5.

Index

African Americans, 40, 108
air bags (in cars), 22, 23–24, 220
air-born germs/chemical toxins
    lead poisoning, 27–28
    mercury poisoning, 28
    plastics/cleaning products, 26
    poop from animals, 2, 29
Alaska Natives, 108
alcoholic beverages
    avoidance, 2, 14, 44–45, 49, 81, 87, 118, 247
    birth defects and, 91
    driving and, 22, 45–46
    facts about, 46
    facts about drinking, 45
    preterm labor and, 110
    stopping before pregnancy, 2
amniotic sac, 140
ankles and feet, swollen, 106
appearance of newborns, 165–166
arm and leg lifts, 22
armpit (axillary) temperature, 237–238
Asian Americans, 40, 108

babies. *See* newborn babies and baby care
baby carrier
    calming influence of, 208, 209
    cloth, 69, 172, 222, 225–226
    flat spot prevention and, 205
    for preemies, 173
    safety factors, 173, 224
    second-hand warning, 72
    stroller *vs.*, 204
baby's growth, pre-birth, 2, 17
back pain (low back pain), 12, 20–21, 140, 144
back sleeping, 214, 215–216, 217
bathing newborns, 168–169, 175–176
bed-sharing, 216–217
biophysical profile (BPP), 120
birth control (contraception)
    after birth of baby, 246, 248–249
    condoms, 25, 105, 249–250
    emergency contraception, 250
    IUD, 250
    partner discussion about, 3
    STD prevention and, 25, 250

birth defects
    age of mother and, 11
    cat poop germs and, 29
    drug use and, 48
    excess vitamin A and, 41
    genetic testing for, 93
    potential causes, 91–92
    prenatal screening, 92
    ultrasound screening, 109
birth of the baby
    delivering the placenta, 142, 150–151
    early delivery, 160–161
    emergence of the baby, 149–150
    epidural/spinal block, 154–155
    episiotomy, 150, 155
    head position surprises, 159
    labor, 140–141, 143, 144–146, 153
    loss of mucus plug, 110, 140
    need for interventions, 152–156
    pain/pain management, 143–144, 153–154
    pushing positions, 149–150
    recovery period, 151–152
    stages of labor, 143
    very fast delivery, 159
    very small baby, 161
birth plan
    birth of the baby, 137–140
    c-section, 158
    episiotomy, 155
    labor, 147–148
    pain management, 153–154
    things to include, 125–127
    third trimester, 118
bleeding gums, 26
blood pressure, 2, 16, 19
    keeping track of, 96–98, 112–114, 129–131, 138
    in older moms, 11
    symptoms of worsening, 120
    third trimester issues, 119–120
bottles
    basics of feeding with, 182–183
    breast milk in, 66, 179, 190, 193
    hand washing before using, 228
    pacifier use and, 189
    supplies for, 68

bras for nursing, 68, 139, 190
Braxton-Hicks contractions, 109, 122, 123
breastfeeding (nursing)
    avoidance of alcohol, drugs, 44, 48, 247
    baby feeding schedule, 186
    basics of, 188
    benefits of, 65–66, 67
    bottle supplementation, 192–193
    discontinuing, 195
    doulas and, 64
    eating right while, 186
    employment and, 29, 67, 192
    expressing milk by hand, 186
    getting ready for, 114
    iodine needs while, 40
    lactation consultant support, 166, 167, 171, 179,
        184–185, 190
    newborn jaundice and, 235
    nipple shape, size, and, 107, 185
    nursing bras and, 68
    nutrition during, 186
    pacifier use and, 69
    positions for holding baby, 187
    provider choice and, 57, 60
    resources, 256, 258, 259, 263
    tips for getting started, 167
    twins/triplets, 189, 247
    WIC program and, 38
breast milk
    alcohol/medicine toxicity and, 44
    benefits of, 65–66
    birth plan inclusion, 126
    bottles of, 192–193
    colostrum (first milk), 186
    expressing method, 186
    medicine toxicity and, 44
    nutritional value, 183
    sharing with other mothers, 189
    twins/triplets and, 189
breasts
    anatomy, 185
    caring for, 190–191, 247
    engorged/painful, 8, 191
breech position babies
    c-section for, 120, 157
    maneuvers for turning baby over, 121
    third trimester possibility, 116
breech tilt maneuver, 121
burn prevention, 223–224
burping, 179, 183, 196

caffeine, 41
car beds, 221
carbohydrates, 35
carbon monoxide detectors, 224
carrying the baby. *See* baby carrier
car safety basics, 22–24, 169–170
car seats
    avoiding second-hand, 72, 226
    buckling baby into, 220
    burn prevention and, 224
    choosing, 70–71, 111, 218
    installing, 219–220
    learning to use, 71
    rear-facing position, 218
    safety basics, 170–171
    sitting up in, 204
    state law requirements, 24, 68
    state laws, 24
    in taxis and buses, 222
    tips, 220–221
cell-free fetal DNA testing, 92
certified nurse midwife (CNM), 56
certified professional midwife (CPM), 56
cervix dilation, 122
cesarean section (C-section)
    for breech position babies, 120
    description, 63, 156–157
    doula support, 64
    elective c-section, 158
    epidural/spinal blocks and, 154–155
    induced labor and, 153
    questions about, 58, 62, 112, 126
    reasons for, 63, 121, 157, 159
    recovery period, 171, 246
    resources, 262
    risk factors, 157–158, 245
    sex after, 248
    vaginal birth after (VBAC), 63, 158
checkups for baby
    kinds of providers, 59
    well-baby checkups, 229–230, 233, 239, 241–242
checkups for mother
    after C-section, 246
    first trimester, 94–98
    prenatal visits, 9, 51, 58, 77
    reasons for, 15–16
    second trimester, 108–109, 112–114
    six-weeks after birth, 248
    talking with provider, 58
    third trimester, 128–135
    vitamin recommendations, 37

children (other than newborn)
  feelings about new baby, 199
  giving attention to, 124
  health history information, 95
  new baby sleep issues, 215, 217
chorionic villus sampling (CVS), 92
circumcision
  choosing, 121
  pros and cons, 170
  recovering from, 174, 175
classes about childbirth, 62
cocaine, 49
colostrum (first milk), 186
comforting newborns, 167, 178–179
condoms, 25, 105, 249–250
constipation management, 107–108
contractions
  amniotic sac breaking and, 140
  Braxton-Hicks, 109, 117, 122, 123
  breathing during, 123, 146, 149
  during exercise, 20
  pain from, 63
  partner support during, 148
  during preterm labor, 110
  timing, 139, 140, 141–142, 144–147
core exercises, 20–22
crawling and climbing, 224–225
crying by baby
  calming strategies, 206, 208–209
  hunger and, 182, 201
  tips for calming mothers, 210
cystic fibrosis (CF) screening, 92

dairy/calcium-rich foods, 36
dental care (oral health), 25–26
diabetes
  gestational (GDM/DM), 108
  post-35 pregnancy concerns, 11
  pre-pregnancy management, 2
  testing for, 108
diaper rash, 174
diapers
  baby's hunger and, 183
  changing, 168–169, 173–174, 201, 208
  checking, 168
  cloth vs. disposable, 68, 186
  feeding and, 182–183
  hand washing after changing, 228
doulas
  advantages of, 64
  choosing, 56
  defined, 10
  new baby care support, 166, 172
  pain control support, 143
  resources, 257
drugs
  during c-section, 63, 157
  dangers to baby, 49
  epidural/spinal block, 154–155
  illegal, avoidance of, 2, 14, 22, 49, 81, 87, 118, 247
  for inducing labor, 153
  miscarriages and, 49, 90
  for pain management, 63, 153–154
  prescription drugs, 48
  preterm labor and, 110
  sleep aids, 154
  strong illegal drugs, 49
due date
  Braxton-Hicks contractions and, 109
  determination of, 3, 9
  late baby, 153
  onset of labor, 140
  prenatal visits and, 58, 120

early labor, 145–147
ear (tympanic) temperature, 238
eating. See feeding newborn babies
e-cigarettes, 46, 248
elective c-section, 158
emotions
  changes during pregnancy, 7, 8
  mixed feelings of partners, 8, 13–14
employment (work)
  breast pump use, 192
  contributions to prenatal care, 10
  insurance benefits and, 52
  maternity leave, 65
  post-baby work, 10, 13
  pregnancy-related issues, 29–30
  support from coworkers, 31
energy drinks, 41
episiotomy
  birth plan inclusion, 126
  caring for, 245
  defined, 57, 150
  pros and cons, 155
exercise
  after baby's birth, 246–247
  benefits, 19
  bridge, 87
  cautions, 20
  charting, 18

exercise (*continued*)
    core exercises, 20–22
    in early labor, 146
    first trimester suggestions, 87
    with friends, 20
    pelvic tilt, 21, 29
    recommendations, 19–22
    in second trimester, 99, 102–104, 106–107
    in third trimester, 118, 123
    walking, 19, 20, 81
expressing breast milk, 186

fall prevention, 222–223
family
    baby care help from, 199–200
    health history knowledge, 3, 91, 93–95, 108
    household care help from, 198, 243
    kangaroo care participation, 178
    mental health issues, 85
    support from, 10, 31, 45, 48, 82–83
family planning, 3, 249–250
family practice doctor, 56, 59
fats, 35, 36
feeding newborn babies, 181–196
    bottle feeding, 193–195
    burping, 179, 183, 196
    gauging baby's fullness, 182–183, 187
    hunger signs, 182
    scheduling, 186
    signs of getting enough milk, 183
    vomiting caution, 183
    See also breastfeeding; breastmilk; formula
fetal alcohol spectrum disorders, 44, 45
fetal gestation, 4 weeks-10 weeks, 2
financial considerations, 10
fish, mercury poisoning from, 28, 42
flat spot (on baby's head) prevention, 204–205
flu shots, 25
folic acid (folate), 2
food and eating (mothers)
    breastfeeding and, 186
    calcium sources, 40
    eating out tips, 37, 38
    healthful habits, 34
    iron and folic acid sources, 39
    omega-3 sources, 39, 40
    preparation safety, 42–43
    raw food warning, 43
    reading food labels, 38
    serving recommendations, 35–36
    snacking during second trimester, 104

    specific nutrient needs, 35
    vegan, vegetarian diets, 36–37, 36=37
    warnings, 28, 41–42
forceps/vacuum extractors, 155–156
forehead temperature, 238
formula
    breastfeeding comparison., 66, 67, 189, 190
    health issues from, 66
    liquid *vs.* powder, 195
    nutritional value, 183
    stool color from, 173
    supplies, 68, 194
    using/choosing, 193–195
friends
    baby care help from, 65, 124, 198, 243
    girls' night out with, 84
    provider suggestions from, 59–60
    second-hand supplies from, 67–68
    sharing with, 14
    smoking considerations, 46–48
    support from, 10, 31, 53, 82–83, 87
    visits during early labor, 146

genital hygiene for newborns, 173
germs and sickness prevention, 25
gestational hypertension, 119
grandparents, 193, 199
Group B streptococcus test, 120
gum and tooth health. *See* oral health

hand washing by caregivers, 26, 28, 228–229
health care providers
    alcohol/smoking information from, 45, 47
    for babies, types of, 59–60
    choosing, 3, 52–58
    defined, 3
    dietary support from, 36–42
    exercise advice from, 19, 20
    miscarriage information from, 12
    paying for, 60
    prenatal visits, 12, 16, 58–59
    support in getting pregnant, 5
    types of, 56–57, 59
    vaccine information from, 25, 31
health of newborn babies
    antibiotic warning, 239
    hand washing by caregivers, 26, 28, 228–229
    medication administration, 239
    newborn jaundice, 235, 236
    newborn screening, 241
    oral health, 40, 176–177, 239–230

RSV virus, 235
  temperature instructions, 235–238
  warning signs, first few months, 236
  well-baby checkups, 229–230, 241–242
heartburn, 105
hemorrhoids management, 107
heroin, 49
Hispanics, 40, 108
hitting baby, avoidance of, 210
homeopathy, 121
home pregnancy tests, 4
hot tubs and saunas, 29
hydration, 205
hygiene tips, 25–26
hypnosis, 121

iodine, 40
IUD (intrauterine device), 250

jaundice in newborns, 235
job-related dangers, 29
journaling, 8, 121

kangaroo care, 178–179
Kegel squeeze exercise, 102–103

labor
  birth team for, 63–64
  contractions, third trimester, 122
  early stage, 145–147
  false *vs.* real, 141
  inducing, 153
  loss of mucus plug, 110, 140
  preparations for, 9
  preterm labor concerns, 109–110
  signs of, 124
  stages of, 42
lactation consultants, 166, 167, 172, 179, 184, 190
lactose intolerance, 40
La Leche League, 184
lead poisoning, 27–28
licensed midwife (LM), 56
listeria/listeriosis, 43
lower back pain, 20–21

maternity leave, 65
Maya Massage, 121
measles, 231
medical marijuana, 48
medication
  antibiotic warnings, 239

avoidance, 54
for baby, 68
breastfeeding and, 184
for circumcised boys, 174
for gestational diabetes, 108
giving to babies, 239
influence on fetal development, 44
keeping track of, 95
medical marijuana, 48
for mood disorders, 251
for new baby's eyes, 164
for pain, 53, 126, 131, 144, 148, 153, 162
pregnancy risks, 3
provider recommendations, 25, 41, 81, 105
toxicity issues, 44
menstrual periods
  baby's growth and, 2
  getting pregnant and, 249
  prepregnancy monitoring, 3
  signs of miscarriage, 90
mercury poisoning, 28, 42
methamphetamine, 49
midwife, 3–5, 52, 55–56
minerals, 35
miscarriages, 89–90
  amniocentesis and, 109
  caffeine and, 41
  drug use and, 49, 90
  first trimester concerns about, 89–91
  lead poisoning and, 27
  listeria and, 43
  in post-35 year old women, 11
  signs of, 11–12, 90
  smoking and, 46
mood swings
  causes of, 83–84, 111, 251
  in partners, 111, 211, 253
  postpartum depression, 250–251
  seeking treatment for, 199
  sleep and, 111, 245, 250–252
  strategies for improving, 84–85, 252
morning sickness, 8
motherhood
  decision-making, 200
  first days, 198
  parents as partners, 198–199
  playing with new baby, 202–205
  talking to new baby, 202
moxibustion, 121
mucus plug, 110, 122, 140
myofascial release, 121

Native Americans, 40, 108
Native Hawaiians, 108
newborn babies and baby care
     appearance, 165–166
     assorted useful items, 69–70
     bathing/cleanliness routine, 168–169, 175–176
     capabilities, 166
     circumcised boy, 174, 175
     clothing choices, 68, 177
     comforting, 167, 178–179
     crying, 208–210
     development, 205–207
     diapers, cloth *vs.* disposable, 68
     doula support, 64
     flat spot prevention, 204–205
     genital hygiene, 173
     going home, 170–171
     health problems' signs, 170
     holding baby, 167, 172–173
     keeping baby warm, 168
     oral health, 40, 176–177, 239–230
     personalities, 201
     playing with, 202–205
     safety basics, 169–170
     second-hand baby gear, 72–73
     skin care, 176
     swaddling, 168
     tummy time for, 203–204, 203–206
newborn jaundice, 235
nursing bras, 68, 139, 190
nursing tank tops, 190
nutrition. *See* feeding newborn babies; food and
     eating (mothers)

obstetrician (OB), 56
omega-3 fatty acids, 39, 40
oral health
     of baby, 40, 176–177, 239–230
     of mother, 18, 25–26, 81
osteopath (DO), 57

Pacific Islanders, 108
pacifiers, 69, 189, 208, 216
pacifier thermometers, 236
pain management
     during baby's birth, 143–144, 153–154
     learning about, 63
     medication for, 53, 126, 131, 144, 148, 153, 162
partner abuse, 88–89
partner tips
     baby care choices, 60

     birth partner choice, 62
     bottle feeding, 196
     breastfeeding, 74, 196
     contractions/labor, 125–127, 146, 148, 151
     exercise, 14
     family planning, 3
     family time, 211
     food habits, 34, 38, 49
     health-related, 4, 31, 240
     lifestyle support, 13–14
     miscarriages, 93
     playing with baby, 211
     post-birth recovery support, 151–152
     preparation for baby, 74, 111
     role of, 4, 6
     safety of baby, 226
     sick baby, 179
     talking about sex, post-birth, 253
paying for baby care, 60
PCP (phencyclidine, Angel dust), 49
pediatricians, 59
pediatric nurse-practitioner, 59
"pelvic tilt" exercise, 21, 29
pertussis (whooping cough) shot (Tdap), 2525
pets, 27
physical health of mother
     air-born germs/chemical toxins, 26–29
     healthy/unhealthy habits checklist, 18
     sources of good advice, 16–17
pica, 41–42
placenta
     anatomy, 78
     c-section and, 157
     delivery of, 142, 150–151
     development, month two, 79–80
     ultrasound exam of, 77
     very fast delivery, 159
Planned Parenthood, 4
playing with new baby, 202–205
positions for breastfeeding, 187
postpartum depression, 250–251
preeclampsia, 119
preemies (premature babies)
     avoiding crowds with, 169
     carrier requirements, 173
     car seat testing for, 221
     clothing choices, 177
     defined, 160
     formula choice, 195
     health problems of, 161
     "kangaroo care" for, 167

sleeping position for, 216
pregnancy
    bodily changes, 8
    emotions during, 7
    first main signs, 4
    preparations, 1–6
    sickness prevention, 25
    teenage, 11
pregnancy, first trimester, 75–98
    birth defect concerns, 91
    bodily changes, 80–81
    checklist to tell providers, 95
    exercise suggestions, 87
    fatigue during, 82
    HIV testing, 91
    miscarriage concerns, 89–91
    month one, 78–79
    month three, 80
    month two, 79
    mood swings, 83–85
    prenatal checkups' components, 94–98
    primary considerations, 77
    quitting alcohol, drugs, tobacco, 87–88
    self-care, 81
    tests during, 92–93
    twins/multiples concerns, 89
    upset stomach, vomiting, 82–83
    weight gain, 85–86
pregnancy, second trimester, 99–114
    Braxton-Hicks contractions, 109
    constipation management, 107–108
    healthy snacking, 104
    heartburn management, 105
    hemorrhoids management, 107
    Kegel squeeze, 102–103
    lifting objects safely, 103
    month five, 100, 113
    month four, 100, 112
    month six, 100–101, 114
    preterm labor concerns, 109–110
    sex during, 104–105, 111
    sitting with knees spread, 104
    squats for core strength, 103
    swollen feet, ankles, 106
    tests during, 108–109
    varicose veins, 106
    walking for exercise, 102
pregnancy, third trimester, 115–136
    baby's kicks and naps, 119
    Braxton-Hicks contractions, 122, 123
    breech position of baby, 120

    exercise suggestions, 118, 123
    final prenatal visits, 122
    healthy habits, 118
    high blood pressure during, 119–120
    home preparedness, 125
    month eight, 116, 117, 130–131
    month nine, 116, 117, 131–135
    month seven, 116, 117, 128–129
    month-to-month checkups, 128–135
    onset of labor, 124
    physical changes, 117
    tests during, 120
    to-do list, 118
    weight gain, 117
pregnancy tests, 4–5
protein, 35

rectal temperature, 237, 238
relaxation strategies, 30
restaurant food tips, 37, 38
Rh (Rhesus) factor test, 108–109
RSV virus in newborns, 235

safe sex, 24–25
safety of baby, 213–226
    bed-sharing risks, 216–217
    burn prevention, 223–224
    car basics, 22–24, 169–170
    fall prevention, 222–223
    home safety, 224–225
    sleep factors, 65, 68, 69, 169, 214–217
seat belts, 22–23
second-hand baby gear, 72–73
second-hand smoke, 46
self-care of mothers, 243–254
    alcohol avoidance, 2, 14, 44, 49, 81, 87, 118, 247
    body healing expectations, 244–247
    breast care, 247
    emergency contraception, 250
    family planning decisions, 249–250
    gentle exercise, 247
    illegal drugs avoidance, 2, 14, 49, 81, 87, 118, 247
    resumption of sex, 248–249
    six-week checkup, 248
    smoking avoidance, 4, 14, 31, 47–49, 87
    stress monitoring, 244
sex
    after birth of baby, 248–249
    due date determination and, 9
    first trimester, 81, 89
    safe sex, 24–25, 105

sex (*continued*)
    second trimester, 104–105, 111
    talking with partner about, 253
    third trimester, 123
sexually transmitted diseases (STDs), 24–25
sexually transmitted infections (STIs), 24–25
shaking baby, avoidance of, 210
shoe recommendations, 29
sleeping pills, 48
sleep of mother
    charting, 18
    during early pregnancy, 82
    during early stage labor, 154
    exercise and, 19
    during later pregnancy, 117
    mood swings and, 111, 245, 250–252
    nursing problems, 190
    post-pregnancy, 243
    strategies for getting, 119
    swollen ankles, feet, and, 106
    when baby sleeps, 164, 172, 198
sleep of newborn baby
    back sleeping, 214, 215–216, 217
    clothing choices, 68
    feeding and, 182–183, 186
    on mother/partner bare chest, 179
    needs of baby, 200–201
    nursing problems, 190
    risk factors, 169, 214–217
    safety factors, 65, 68, 69, 169, 214–217
    strategies for getting, 207–208, 211
    tummy sleeping, 215–216
smoke alarms, 224
smoking
    avoidance, 4, 14, 31, 47–49, 87
    hand washing after, 228
    miscarriages/stillbirths risks, 46
    preterm labor and, 110
    sleeping safety and, 216
    tips for quitting, 47–48
stillbirths, 11, 108
stockings, elastic, 29
stretching exercises, 19
Sudden Infant Death Syndrome (SIDS), 169, 213
suffocation during sleep (of new baby), 169
swimming, 19

talking to new baby, 202
teenage pregnancy, 11
temperature, instructions for taking, 235–238
thermometers, types of, 236–238

throwing baby, avoidance of, 210
tooth and gum health, 25–26
toxemia, 119
"triple screen" (fist trimester), 92
tummy sleeping, 215–216
tummy time for new babies, 203–204, 203–206
twins
    breastfeeding, 189, 247
    kangaroo care for, 178
    partner support with, 200
    premature potential, 160
    preterm labor and, 128
    risk factors, 89
    ultrasound confirmation, 92
    weight gain with, 86

umbilical cord
    anatomy, 78, 79
    care of, 174
    c-section and, 157
    cutting, 150
    drug use and, 48
    infection of, 236

vaccines
    diseases prevented by, 232–233
    for mothers, 25, 31
    questions about, 232–233
    reasons for getting, 230–231
    recommendations by age 2, 234
    record card, 230
    timing of, 216, 229, 231–232
vaginal birth after cesarean (VBAC), 63, 158
varicose veins, 106
vegan/vegetarian diets, 36–37
vitamins and minerals
    calcium, 40
    folate (folic acid), 2, 39
    iodine, 40
    iron, 39
    omega-3 fatty acids, DHA, 39, 40
    prenatal needs, 39
    vitamin A, 41
vomiting. *See* morning sickness

walking, 19, 20, 81
Webster Technique (chiropractic care), 121
well-baby checkups, 229–230, 241–242
Women, Infants, and Children Program (WIC), 38

yoga, prenatal, 20